Beyond The Reluctant Move

A Practical Approach to Emotional Wellbeing in Residential Aged Care Facilities

Dr Julie Bajic Smith (PhD)

First published by Ultimate World Publishing 2020
Copyright © 2020 Dr Julie Bajic Smith

ISBN

Paperback - 978-1-922372-08-6
Ebook - 978-1-922372-09-3

Cover design: Ultimate World Publishing
Layout and typesetting: Ultimate World Publishing
Editor: Marinda Wilkinson
Cover Photo: GagliardiPhotography-Shutterstock.com

ULTIMATE WORLD
PUBLISHING

Ultimate World Publishing
Diamond Creek,
Victoria Australia 3089
www.writeabook.com.au

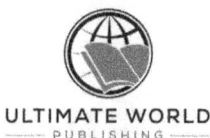

Dedication

For my children,
Hazel and Henry,
and in memory of my grandparents.

Contents

Dedication   iii

Foreword   vii

Introduction   ix

Part I: Emotional Wellbeing in Late Life..............................**1**

Chapter 1: Late Life Changes   3

Chapter 2: The Big Move   15

Chapter 3: Wellbeing Factors   25

Chapter 4: Common Mental Health Conditions
in Late Life   35

Part II: Identifying Strengths..**47**

Chapter 5: All Is Not Lost   49

Chapter 6: Always Learning   61

Part III: Establishing Social Goals **73**

Chapter 7: Goal Setting   75

Part IV: Resilience Boosting Activities **91**

Chapter 8: Onsite Activities   93

Chapter 9: Sharing Memories   111

Part V: Integrated Collaboration **121**

Chapter 10: Building Support Networks   123

Chapter 11: Involving Families   133

Chapter 12: Psychological Wellbeing
 for the Workforce   141

References   149

Appendices   155

Acknowledgements   171

Foreword

'If you don't like something change it; if you can't change it, change the way you think about it.'

Mary Engelbreit

A powerful quote – however, it is easier said than done. Moving into an aged care facility is often the final step after all avenues to keep an older person in their own home have been exhausted. Sometimes there are long waitlists to move into a facility, other times the entire process can feel fast and rushed. Either way, in most cases, once an individual moves into an aged care facility they rarely move back home.

Accepting the move can be difficult, as the older person needs to become familiar with their new environment, learn routines, accept external support with personal care needs and adjust to a new way of interacting with their loved ones, which is no longer characterised with care delivery and support in their own home. These changes can impact an older person's emotional wellbeing and that of those who support them. And, we have not even touched on the older person's health status and changes that may have occurred in their physical abilities or cognitive functioning.

Recognising how to best support an older person and help with the adjustment is important, but it is not always straightforward, and relatives and staff may feel stuck for what to say and do. Certain topics may be avoided, distraction techniques used and isolation and withdrawal normalised.

Over the last decade I have watched the prevalence of mental health conditions in this population slowly rise. In 2018, depression was the most commonly diagnosed mental health condition among people in permanent residential aged care (Australian Institute of Health and Welfare [AIHW], 2019).

Open conversations, preventions, early detection and non-pharmacological strategies are vital in minimising the prevalence of mental health conditions in older adults in residential care. I strongly believe that every older person in residential aged care deserves to be heard, understood and loved. This book is for anyone who supports older people and needs practical wellbeing tips which they can implement today.

The elderly have their voice too – hear them out!

Julie Bajic Smith
Sydney 2020

Introduction

'*Mum, we are going out for lunch,*' said Helen to her elderly mother Gwen one morning. She was anxiously preparing for her mother to enter residential care that afternoon. Helen felt scared, nervous, yet quietly relieved that Gwen would finally be getting the right level of care, as she was not coping well at home and had already had several falls. The only problem was that she did not know how to tell her mum the plan, as she knew that her mum did not want to leave her home. Gwen was fiercely independent and reluctant to accept her declining physical health, even arguing with her doctor and the geriatrician about her ability to remain living independently. She was adamant she could cope on her own, despite her recent falls which required hospitalisation. Gwen would angrily tell Helen, '*For heaven sake, look at the world today, I am safest right here in my own home*'. Adding to Helen's concern was the feedback from the home care workers, who called in a couple of times a week and helped Gwen with shopping. The workers were concerned about Gwen's health too, her reduced mobility, as well as the impact of isolation on her health.

After lunch, Helen dropped Gwen off at a local, newly refurbished aged care hostel and told her she would stay '*for a night, as requested by the doctor'*. She eventually told Gwen that she would not be able to return to her home, as she is no longer safe to live on her own. To help with the packing, Helen arranged for Gwen's furniture to be distributed among the family and called a charity to take a significant proportion of Gwen's belongings. Helen only wanted the best for Gwen. Gwen in turn felt rejected, betrayed and upset.

Fortunately, most older adults are in good health and maintain their independence well into their twilight years. Older adults are, in general, happier than younger adults. They are satisfied with family relationships, have meaningful social and recreational involvements and are more emotionally and interpersonally adaptable than younger adults. However, those who have declining physical and cognitive health are more likely to feel isolated, withdrawn and experience depression and/or anxiety. Many of us are uncomfortable broaching the subject of the future with a loved one whose health is declining yet may feel overwhelmed with the responsibilities of day-to-day care.

According to the AIHW, about five percent of older Australians currently live in residential care, with the numbers continually increasing with our demographics and ageing population. Supported accommodation has many negative connotations, despite the increasing trend of low care facilities, such as hostels, which promote independence, outings and social support. Many older adults who move into a hostel experience improved health due to better nutrition, regular exercise and increased socialisation. However, discussing the transition can be difficult, particularly if the person has an impaired perception of independence and is putting themselves at risk of physical harm and emotional withdrawal, due to limited social support.

Beyond the Reluctant Move was written in consultation with aged care experts, facility managers, allied health professionals, diversional therapists, recreational activity officers, personal care staff, registered nurses and, most importantly, with older adults who entered residential care and their families and friends. The aim of the book is to dispel the common myths associated with the transition into residential care and help you consider the needs for each individual, regardless of their health status or life stage. Through evidence-based tips, practical strategies and guidance, you'll learn how to openly communicate and assist older adults to make a successful transition into care when the time is right.

Moving into residential care is challenging – but access to the right information and helpful tips from others who have already made the move themselves can enormously assist with the process. You are not alone. Many families report a sense of relief once a loved one enters residential care, as they are receiving the right level of support for their needs and are in the appropriate place for the amount of care needed.

Unfortunately, a lot of people think it is normal to get depressed as you get old – and that it is even more normal to experience cognitive changes, most notably dementia. Some research has even revealed that doctors often overlook mental health in the aged and fail to diagnose and treat it (Uncapher & Arean, 2000). This trend has significant implications for the older person, and for those who support them, as it may mean that the level of support needed is higher as the individual's mental health has not been addressed. If an older person has symptoms of depression and is reluctant to engage in physical activities, they are more likely to experience changes in their mobility, be at a greater risk of falls and experience isolation.

In the chapters that follow, we disentangle the issues that arise for older people when they move into residential care. How can the process be managed better to ensure a smooth transition and adjustment to the new environment? What is the role of families in supporting the elderly and how can they help their loved one adjust? There are many different approaches that can be implemented, and the focus of this book is to share simple and effective strategies and practical tips that can help anyone who works in aged care or supports an older person in an aged care setting.

Humans are social creatures with emotional needs for relationships and positive connections to others. Humans are not meant to survive, let alone thrive, in isolation. Therefore, when individuals find themselves isolated, due to changes in their health status or support network, it is important to look at ways their connections can be enhanced, as it is the key to improving emotional wellbeing. Human connection includes conversations taking place face-to-face, the tone of voice being heard, facial expressions seen and energy being felt. Phone calls and video calls have their place, but nothing can beat the stress-busting, mood-boosting power of quality face-to-face time with other people.

Creating emotionally supportive and healthy aged care environments is not a process completed in isolation by health professionals. Emotionally insightful aged care providers are not 10 times more funded, 10 times more experienced or 10 times more staffed. The approach has nothing to do with the size of the provider, it has everything to do with five skills that make an organisation stand out from the rest and lead the industry in raising the bar to improve emotional wellbeing in their residents.

This book is underpinned with five skills that emotionally aware aged care providers focus on, which are:

- Emotional Wellbeing
- Identifying Strengths
- Establishing Social Goals
- Resilience Boosting Activities
- Integrated Collaboration

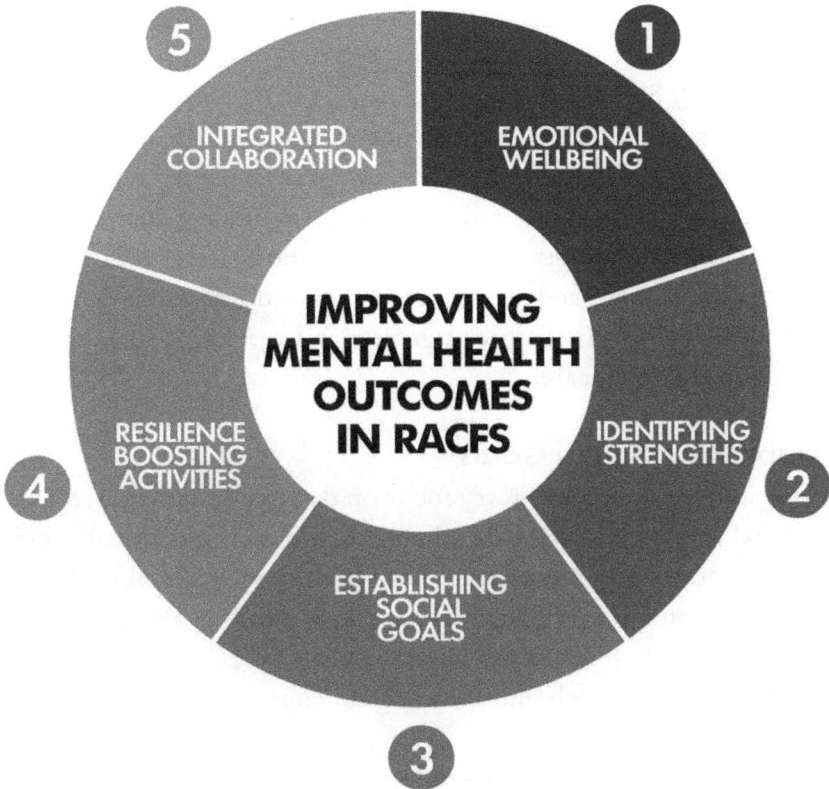

Emotional Wellbeing

Emotionally aware aged care providers have a screening process to check the wellbeing of their residents down pat. They have good systems in place to review admissions and to escalate concerns to health professionals for any residents who appear to have ongoing difficulty adjusting to the new environment. This does not mean that they just tick the box and await feedback from health professionals – instead, they continue to work with the individual to identify ways the older person's emotional wellbeing can be nurtured, such as providing opportunities for one on one time and implementing reflective listening. If the provider does not have a clear system in place for resident reviews and escalation of concerns, they cannot measure progress.

Identifying Strengths

Resilience and confidence grows when we focus on the strengths, not the weaknesses of older adults. They do not need regular reminders of activities they are no longer able to complete independently, such as accessing the community, driving, going to the beach or bushwalking. Emotionally aware aged care providers are innovators in identifying individual strengths which can greatly assist older people adjust to living in residential care.

Establishing Social Goals

It's no longer enough to simply focus on day-to-day activities, it's also essential to plan activities ahead and review each individual's social goals. Emotionally aware aged care providers assist older people to develop and achieve their unique individual goals. They work collaboratively to help clients maintain those goals, ensuring the lives of older people are rich, meaningful and engaged.

Resilience Boosting Activities

Emotionally aware aged care providers intrinsically understand the types of activities that boost wellbeing in older adults in care and offer these activities on a regular basis. Each activity is evaluated and its effectiveness is measured. This does not necessarily mean that activities are more expensive, time consuming or demanding, they are simply better ways to provide engagement and fulfillment in residents.

Integrated Collaboration

Emotionally aware aged care providers do not work in isolation. They collaborate with families, internal multidisciplinary teams, external providers and health professionals to achieve the best outcomes for their residents.

Looking closely at a number of providers who apply this approach, it can be noted they are consistently in the upper bracket of their field. It does not take years, it does not take luck and it does not necessarily take hard work. It is about focusing on the things that matter most – the emotional wellbeing of residents.

Part I

Emotional Wellbeing in Late Life

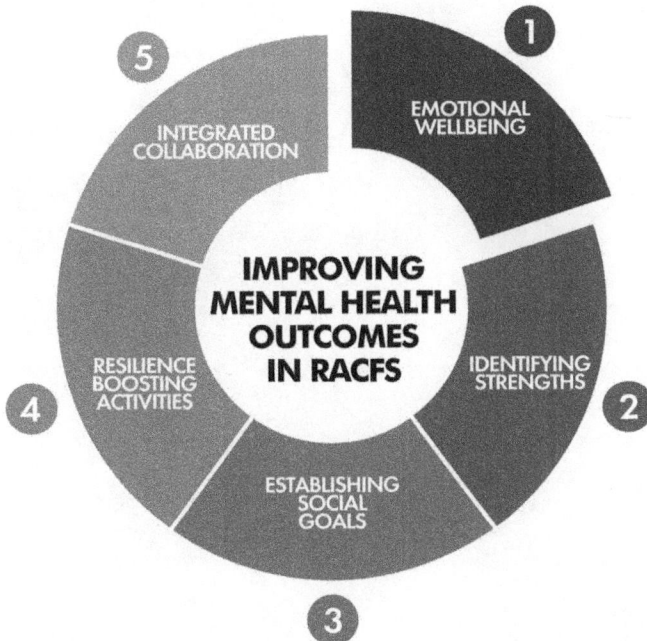

5 INTEGRATED COLLABORATION

1 EMOTIONAL WELLBEING

IMPROVING MENTAL HEALTH OUTCOMES IN RACFS

2 IDENTIFYING STRENGTHS

4 RESILIENCE BOOSTING ACTIVITIES

3 ESTABLISHING SOCIAL GOALS

CHAPTER 1

Late Life Changes

To be old and wise; what a privilege denied to many. Of course, with positive ageing comes a number of rewarding benefits, such as sharing special memories with loved ones and being able to travel. Then again, there can be some challenges, such as reduced endurance, a higher risk of sensory impairment, no longer driving and an increased need for support.

The last century has seen many medical advances and scientific findings on how to improve our physical health and wellbeing. We now better understand the relationship between physical activity, dietary intake and social connection, and how this impacts our wellbeing and longevity. We no longer attribute all the negative effects of our poor health outcomes on genetics and better understand the role we all play in our own health. The food we eat can either be the safest and most powerful form of medicine or the slowest form of poison. However, not everyone who enters late life requires nor receives support. In fact, most older adults remain fairly independent, sometimes even caring for others, until their death. For some, the need for an increased level of support may arise in mid-life, such as diagnosis of early onset dementia. For others, it may happen later in life following the death of a spouse, falls or poor mobility. If in-home support is not available, or has been exhausted, these health changes may result in admission to residential care, a process that's not often discussed or favourably looked upon.

In the period between 2017–2018, the aged care sector provided services to over 1.3 million Australians. Almost 1 million individuals received support in their own homes, and about 300,000 received support in residential care. The average age on admission to permanent residential aged care was 82 years for men and 84 years for women. Many of those admitted to residential care had previously received a home care package, which included government subsidised support for daily living activities (AIHW, 2019).

There is often the assumption that older people become automatically eligible for residential care, based on their age alone. However, the admission is met with stringent eligibility criteria following a formal assessment by an independent assessor relying on medical evidence and a review of daily living activities in the older person's home. Subsequently, there are various reasons for admission into residential care, including frailty, significant cognitive decline, mental health support needs and exhaustion of home care services due to declining health status. Once admitted to residential care, the average length of stay for a permanent resident in residential care is around two years, and women tend to stay longer than men. Some residents move to another facility, some move back home (which is rare but still possible), but most stay at the facility until their death.

Late life changes do not always occur slowly, such as the gradual decline in mobility and sensory impairment. Sometimes they can be quite sudden. Betty, aged 94, was walking to an art exhibition in downtown Sydney, when she suddenly slipped and heard a little 'crack'. Betty was determined she was fine, but passers-by called the ambulance and she was transported to a hospital where she was diagnosed with a hip fracture which required surgery. Betty never again laid eyes on her immaculate two-bedroom apartment which she called home for over four decades. The stairs in her rustic building prevented safe access and subsequently Betty's family decided the best option was for Betty to move to an aged care facility. This decision is one that Betty has never fully accepted and she still holds some resentment with her family, which she has been working hard to put behind her.

Understanding Emotional Wellbeing in Late Life

The vast majority of older adults enjoy better mental health than younger people. They are resilient, financially secure and less stressed than the working population. Many engage in vocational activities, such as paid employment and volunteer work, travel, hobbies and sports. However, challenges tend to arise when the older person experiences health setbacks, which may affect their ability to maintain social engagement and attend to the activities of daily living. These experiences can affect an older person's confidence, emotional wellbeing and view of themselves and their abilities. Although many people age without significant changes to their own health, they are likely to experience inevitable changes around them. This may include, more frequent grief and loss in late life, such as the death of their spouse, siblings, friends and acquaintances. Cessation of driving and the subsequent reduced access to their local community and social interactions can have an accumulative effect on their wellbeing, as can the side effects of medication, chronic pain and reduced mobility. The more isolated the older person feels the more likely they are to experience changes in their emotional wellbeing. Older people may become more reliant on their children and relatives to attend to daily activities and social interactions. This can assist in reducing the older person's isolation and wellbeing, however, the increased need for support may put strains or carers, stretching their commitments and ability to provide support on an ongoing basis.

Historically, our understanding of the emotional needs of older people has been predominately based around those who live in their own homes. Research studies examining factors associated with wellbeing in late life and have found that many older people do not seek support for their emotional wellbeing (Bagley et al., 2000; Davison et al., 2012; Eyers et al., 2012). Stigma, ageism and the lack of mental health professionals who specialise in supporting this age group are some of the contributing factors of this trend. In residential care, the access to mental health professionals is even more limited, as there are very few organisations who employ mental health professionals and many external providers are not experienced in conducting clinical work outside of their consulting rooms. On top of this, limited funding for mental health support results in out-of-pocket expense for the older person which can further hinder service accessibility. Aged care providers then find themselves in a position where they have residents who are isolated, withdrawn, emotionally distressed and reluctant to participate in activities on offer at the facility.

However, the transition to residential care is not always a negative experience and one that triggers negative changes to emotional wellbeing. For some, it can mean better social connection, more access to nursing support, improved physical activity, social engagement and access to hot meals and warm showers. In those instances, residents may have been exposed to an unsuitable environment prior to admission into residential care. There may have been a history of social isolation, neglect or even elder abuse. These examples highlight the importance of skilful support and guidance prior to, and on the day of, admission. The first few days in the new environment need to be carefully managed with a balance between alone time and encouragement for social engagement which can assist in boosting the overall health and wellbeing of an older person. Older people who are well supported during the admission may be faster to adjust to the new environment and be more willing to engage in activities and form new friendships.

Statistics on an Ageing Population

Statistics from the World Health Organisation reminds us that with increasing age, numerous underlying physiological changes occur, and the risk of chronic disease rises. By age 60, the major burdens of disability and death arise from age-related losses in hearing, seeing and moving, and noncommunicable diseases, including heart disease, stroke, chronic respiratory disorders, cancer and dementia (World Health Organisation [WHO], 2011). However, the presence of these health conditions says nothing about the impact they may have on an older person's life. There is a significant difference between individuals and how they respond to changes in their physical health and emotional wellbeing.

In Australia, the population of people aged 65 and over has increased significantly in the last 100 years and is predicted to continue growing. In 1901, the proportion of people aged 65 years and over represented 4% of population, in 2011 the same age bracket represented 14% of the population and in 2101 it is predicted that people aged 65 plus will represent 25% of the population (AIHW, 2019). This significant growth is resulting in increasing demand for services and awareness of the needs of older people. Statistically, only about 5% of older adults will move into an aged care facility. In 2019, that percentage is almost 300,000 individuals.

Onset of Mental Health Conditions

In defining mental health conditions, it is crucial to distinguish the language used, address negative stigma and have a better understanding of labels used. Often terms can be thrown around which can be misrepresentative and hurtful.

So how do we define the difference between mental health and mental illness? Easy – every person needs to have good mental health and resilience when faced with the challenges of daily life. However, our mental health can decline for various reasons and affect our wellbeing. For some individuals, they may have been first diagnosed with a mental health condition in early life, which is defined as early onset, whereas others may not have had any significant emotional disturbances until late life, which is defined as late onset mental health condition(s).

For individuals diagnosed with early onset of mental health conditions, genetic factors and life experiences can contribute to an increased risk of developing a chronic serious mental illness, such as schizophrenia and bipolar disorder. Whilst the purpose of this book is not to examine chronic serious mental illness in early life, it is important to recognise the role of such experiences in late life and how they affect individuals in residential care. Individuals with chronic serious mental illness often have higher risk factors for developing mild cognitive impairment, are more frequently single and come from lower socio-economic backgrounds. These individuals are likely to age prematurely with high rates of obesity, vascular disease, diabetes and have a history of alcohol and drug misuse. Some of these factors, such as a history of bipolar disorder or depression, may be a risk factor for dementia in late life and these individuals are more likely to require maintenance psychotropic medication.

Late onset mental health disorders include depression, anxiety, bipolar disorder, late life psychoses and alcohol/drug misuse.

These conditions often have organic, in particular neurological factors in their presentation as well as psychosocial factors, which can include financial status, support networks and physical health. Late onset mental health disorders can be associated with mild cognitive impairment, and without professional mental health support and thorough assessment (including discussion with family and relatives), it can be difficult to establish if the cause for cognitive impairment is due to a mental health condition or early symptoms of dementia. Typically, individuals with late onset mental health disorders are more likely to have family supports and have reasonable socio-economical background than those with early onset disorder.

Cognitive Decline in Old Age

Many older people fear experiencing cognitive decline such as dementia in late life and often seek support from health professionals in how to enhance their memory. Those who experience mild cognitive changes may not have insight into their impairment. This can result in short-term memory loss including repetition, forgetfulness around routine and getting lost. There are a number of reasons for cognitive changes in late life and dementia is just one of them. Diagnosis of dementia can have a significant emotional effect on the individual and their family, while for others it can be a sense of relief to finally know the cause of the symptoms. Other reasons for cognitive changes may include emotional status, side effects of medication, disruption in routine and sleep deprivation.

Cognitive decline due to emotional changes can be reversed and outcomes can be improved – but not treating emotional changes which may be due to mental health conditions can have serious consequences for the older person and their physical health.

The effect of untreated mental health conditions includes:

- reduced quality of life
- unnecessary suffering for the older person
- increased burden for the family and service provider
- social and economic impact as the person requires more care and support
- increased use of health services
- increased physical morbidity
- increased risk of mortality and suicide.

These effects are significant and there are a number of ways in which addressing the mental health needs of this population is important, as outlined in later chapters.

Cognitive decline due to a neurological condition, such as dementia, is far less likely to reverse and improve, however, with a structured routine the effects can be slowed down. In a 2001 study, researchers examined memory in almost 900 individuals aged 70 to 93 years. The study found that crystallised abilities (factual information such as age, family dynamics and information about major life achievements), remained largely intact, but that cognitive speed and memory performance tended to decline with age (Christensen, 2001).

It is normal to experience some cognitive decline in older age, for example, taking longer to recall information or remember some details. However, the presence of dementia in old age is not a normal part of ageing. Prevalence rates for dementia across the world are relatively low, being only around 5–8% of the population aged 60 and over (WHO, 2017), with the risks increasing with age. For adults aged 70–74 the prevalence of dementia is only 1–3%, however, the prevalence of dementia increases to 10–21% for adults aged above 85 years (Hendersen et al., 1994).

Medical Comorbidity

Medical comorbidity refers to experiencing multiple health problems at the same time. Common comorbidities in late life include arthritis, hypertension, reduced visual acuity, hearing impairment, diabetes and cardiovascular disease. Changes in emotional wellbeing can be caused by changes in physical health status, for example, if an older person had a stroke or reduced fine motor skills due to arthritis, their ability to engage in recreational activities may be impaired and this can affect how they feel. Similarly, emotional wellbeing can also affect physical health. Those who feel sad or down may be less inclined to exercise and keep active, which can then affect their physical bodies and (in late life in particular) may reduce mobility.

One of the most common comorbidities for an older person in a residential setting is presenting with symptoms of depression and cognitive impairment. It can be difficult to establish the primary disorder – did the person first experience changes in their mood or in their memory? At times, it can be changes in mood and reduced activity levels which can affect memory, particularly if the older person is isolated and not regularly engaging in interpersonal activities and interactions. On the other hand, for some individuals who first experience cognitive changes, depression can come secondary, particularly if they have insight into their memory changes and this affects their confidence and self-esteem. Many older people with early cognitive changes report feeling ashamed that their memory is not as good as it used to be. They can also experience grief and loss, as their future and prospects have changed and they are now facing a different life path to the one they envisioned.

Loneliness

Loneliness refers to the discrepancy between the number and quality of the relationships that an individual wants and those they actually have. Some individuals only have two friends, but if those friendships are deep, meaningful and meet the all their needs, then they are not lonely. Others could be in a crowd of people and feel lonely, as they do not meaningfully relate or connect to any of those individuals. Loneliness is common in residential care, especially if residents are not encouraged to socialise and interact or if during the initial settlement period their solitude and withdrawal is normalised and accepted as a personality trait.

Loneliness is a common condition affecting around one in three adults (Eyers et al., 2012). It affects people of all ages and is particularly common in adults who find it difficult to interact with others due to declining physical health and sensory impairment. The effects of loneliness are widespread. Research indicates that loneliness can damage our brain, compromise our immune system, and lead to depression and suicide (Eyers et al., 2012). Loneliness has also been found to increase the risk of dying prematurely, and it can be as detrimental to our health as smoking 15 cigarettes a day (Tiwari, 2013). Individuals who experience loneliness tend to feel more tired, even if they get sufficient sleep, and feel stressed in situations that others cope better in. This has been attributed to the effects of reduced interactions with others and the lack of access to connect with others to problem-solve issues on a day-to-day basis.

Interestingly, loneliness is not just about how individuals feel but reflects also on their behaviours. In older people this can include changes in eating patterns, skipping meals and opting for less healthy options, due to lack of motivation to prepare a healthy and fulfilling meal. Individuals who experience loneliness in a residential setting are also less likely to engage in activities such as exercise and group activities, which are important for physical and mental health. They may feel uncomfortable and unfamiliar in the environment and be self-conscious of their efforts, not wanting to put themselves in situations where they may get embarrassed if they say or do something incorrectly and are perceived as being 'silly' or 'stupid'.

It is easy to assume that the best way to overcome loneliness is to simply talk to a few more people or to put complete strangers in the same environment and presume they will become the best of friends and overcome their loneliness. These strategies can help, but will not necessarily result in the formation of meaningful relationships. However, the addition of an experienced facilitator who can make introductions and start discussions based on common interests can be highly beneficial. In residential care the addition of careful planning of reminiscence activities, skill-building activities as well as strength-based programs which focus on the resident's abilities rather than losses can also help.

When people become lonely, they can start to act and see the world differently. They may begin to notice the threats in their environment more readily, expect to be rejected more often and become more judgemental of the people they interact with. People they talk to can feel this, and as a result, it can drive them away, which further perpetuates their loneliness cycle.

Better interactions can be formed by starting a discussion asking the older person about their pleasant memories, such as favourite holidays and family traditions, rather than talking about the reasons for admission to aged care and the help and support they require. The facilitator will also need to be mindful of sensory impairment and incorporating written cues into the program. In the Be Well Group Program this is accommodated with scripts for each session. More details about this program can be found at the end of the book.

DIGGING DEEP

1. What are some of the common misconceptions about ageing introduced to you by your parents, teachers or elderly family members when you were growing up?

2. Do you ever notice yourself making similar misconceptions in your day-to-day conversations? For example, if you are a parent, do you share those misconceptions with your children? Do you say them to your friends?

3. When you reflect on your life and key older people that inspired you, what characteristics did those people have? What set them apart from others their age?

CHAPTER 2

The Big Move

Do not say the 'N' word! We will not talk about that. Nursing homes, residential aged care facilities, homes or even 'old people's prisons' as described by some clients over the years, do not necessarily have warm or positive connotations associated with them. As many older people have shared during individual and group sessions, they could never foresee themselves living in those environments prior to the move and they pitied those whose circumstances brought them there. However, if the older person's health significantly declines and the possibility of moving to a residential aged care facility has not been discussed, it may hinder the adjustment. *'But, I should stay at home,'* – yes, ideally the older person should stay living where they wish, but this is not always possible or sustainable if their health is compromised and significantly affects activities of daily living. Avoiding the topic of the prospect of moving into an aged care facility can affect the wellbeing of the older person, cause tension in families, result in more difficult adjustment and create challenging dynamics for facilities to manage. There have been several instances where families have asked for a psychologist to break the news to their loved one about moving into care, or they have resorted to telling their relative that they are going to stay in a hotel. This has not been successful.

Krystina was a Polish migrant, a retired psychology professor, who was referred for a psychological review due to 'challenging behaviours'. Nursing home staff described her as being rude, often demanding of services and demeaning towards staff and other residents. Krystina suffered a stroke in her tiny unit on the north shore of Sydney. She managed to call an ambulance and after extensive hospitalisation and rehabilitation, she has never returned to the unit, as climbing two sets of stairs was not possible with her walking frame and in her frail state. Krystina reported feeling angry and frustrated with her predicament, particularly as she has experienced unfathomable personal loss in her early life in Poland during WWII. Since the age of 17, she has been the only remaining member of her family with both of her parents and siblings killed. Krystina was initially cold and distant during the meeting but eventually warmed up and asked to see 'that psychologist' again. Over the course of a couple of weeks she became well engaged in psychological services to the point of not only attending group sessions but gathering other residents to attend. In group sessions, she often spoke about the importance of not only discussing positive ageing, but also acknowledging the difficulties experienced with 'negative ageing' which includes moving into an aged care facility.

Moving into an aged care facility is not always a setback. Some individuals thrive in a residential setting, as they feel less isolated, experience increased appetite, receive more frequent personal care and feel more connected to others. Subsequently, individuals can maintain a healthy weight, increase physical tolerance with regular exercise and physiotherapy as well as improve their outlook on life, having made new friendships and connections. On the other hand, the move can be difficult for some, particularly those whose circumstances changed suddenly. There is no easy pattern or step-by-step guide to follow when moving into residential care and how to best accept the change. Every person's journey is unique and characterised by their own health circumstances, insight into personal and social care supports, availability of emotional support, financial position and geographical location. Often what connects people to one another is not their losses and reasons for admission to care, but rather their interests, passion and outlook on life.

Families play an integral role when it comes to supporting the older person's move into care. Families are involved in researching facilities, facilitating the move and advocating on behalf of their loved ones. Families also often have their own process of accepting what has occurred and grieving the loss of the relationship and future that they anticipated for their loved one. This could be a wife who has great difficulty accepting that her 70-year-old husband has been diagnosed with dementia and that they can no longer plan driving trips together or enjoy their retirement at home, or a daughter whose mother is experiencing a number of falls and is no longer able to live on her own. It can be difficult to decide and accept that an aged care home is the best solution for the older person, as family may feel a lot of negative connotation associated with the environment and at times a sense of guilt or shame. This is why it is important to ensure that family is also supported through the process and included in collaboration and planning care needs as well as given opportunities to get support for their own grief and loss.

Slow Growers

When late life health changes occur slowly over a long period of time these changes are described as slow growers. These are often subtle changes that occur gradually, including empty nesting, retirement, transitioning from our current role in society and in family (for example, a spouse taking on additional caring roles and duties), changes in our five senses and slowing down in movement. These changes are defined as 'role losses' and may result in symptoms of anxiety or depression due to the functional importance given to certain roles which serve to maintain one's positive self-image and identity (Feldman, 1994). The cognitive and emotional changes an older person experiences may become more evident to relatives, such a repetition of information or neglect in grooming and eating habits. In those instances it can be difficult to draw a line in the sand when to determine that the older person firstly requires help with those tasks, and from there evaluate if they are able to remain living independently.

At a family workshop a daughter of a resident shared her experience: *'Mum had no insight into her own deterioration which made the resistance to moving into a home even greater. It was recommended by the doctor that Mum move into care but trying to explain this to her was difficult. It was hard to explain that we were no longer able to give her the care she needed.'*

In those instances, families may have better insight into the support the older person requires, but the older person themselves may not have the insight or feel ready to move into care. If the older person is currently receiving support, they may not have an insight into the extent of that support and what would happen if it was no longer available.

The main consideration when reviewing independence in older people who experience slow changes in their memory or functioning is the risk involved in staying in their own home. If the older person is exposed to high safety risks, such as leaving kitchen appliances on or getting lost in the community, then independent living may not be sustainable for much longer. If, on the other hand the symptoms are relatively mild and they have good support at home then it may be possible for the older person to remain living in their own home. There are many individuals with mild cognitive changes who live in retirement villages where they are well supported by their local community and they may also receive in-home support.

Another relative shared, *'The biggest challenge was getting Mum to agree to move into care. She had always said she didn't want to be a burden, but that was years before she had dementia. She has always pitied anyone in "a home".'*

The above reflection highlights the personality changes that may occur in the older person as a result of cognitive impairment. The person may become more determined about their independence due to the lack of insight into the extent of their impairment. They may become angry, frustrated and frightened of their future.

Sudden Changes

In some instances, the older person's level of support needs can change suddenly. One day they may be fully independent, to the extent that they are in fact caring for someone else, and the next day they are the ones who require care and support. In those cases, adjustment into an aged care facility can be more difficult, as the individual experiences a greater sense of loss and acceptance of the rather traumatic set of events which led to their sudden change in environment and support needs. Those individuals may require additional support from health professionals, family and friends through this difficult time.

'I remember the date quite clearly, it was the 10/10. I was home in bed and suddenly I was overwhelmed with this strange sensation in my body. I knew it was a stroke. My husband called the ambulance and I have never been home again. My life as I knew it was over. There is no way I want to see my house again. I don't think I could handle it. I was caring for my husband and suddenly I became the one that needs support. It's hard. My stroke has done so much damage — I can't

walk, write or do any fine motor skill tasks with my right hand. I am in an aged care facility and wake up next to my roommate, not my husband. It is terrible. I know I should think about the glass being half full, but my complete life is the empty part missing in that glass.'

Individuals who experience sudden changes in their health need to be offered opportunities to grieve openly and discuss the impact of their health setbacks with others. Not allowing those opportunities can cause further distress for the individual. They may not always require a mental health professional to intervene, particularly in the early weeks and months of the event. Good listening skills from others are important, allowing the older person to share the impact of their loss and offering simple steps in promoting wellness, such as spending time outdoors or in nature (if possible), which can be therapeutically beneficial. This is also an opportunity to remind the older person of their strengths and resilience, the skills which they still hold and are able to use to get through challenges.

Advice from Other Families

Many families over the years have reported how they struggled to find useful information when their loved one was moving into care. This includes information on how to organise the transition into an aged care facility, the frequency of visits and type of activities during the visits. There are no fast and easy solutions to these questions, as the recommendations depend on the older person, the relative and their relationship.

At a workshop. one relative stated, *'The best advice given to me was to choose a home that was closest to my home'.*

They explained that this was beneficial as they could attend more frequently and come in at short notice. This advice may not work for everyone, as perhaps being too close may encourage more frequent visits which may impact the older person's adjustment to the environment – they would be sitting and waiting for their relative to attend instead of joining in with onsite activities.

Therefore, it was not surprising to hear another relative say how she received advice about the importance of looking after herself and letting their relative settle into the new environment by trusting staff: *'Don't visit too often. It's like when your five-year-old starts school. Go and have a coffee and a cry.'*

A common concern for many relatives is the impact of their loved one's diminishing memory. In some instances, memory impairment is due to emotional wellbeing, in others it is due to neurological conditions such as stroke and dementia.

Some relatives reach out to organisations, such as Dementia Australia to learn how to improve communication with their loved one: *'The most helpful advice was about how to communicate with someone with dementia. It is a difficult skill to acquire as it is hard to learn to put aside personal emotions. It's almost like learning a new language.'*

From these examples it is evident that loved ones embark on a new journey when their relatives move into care, learning more about health conditions, the impact on the individual and how to enhance their connection.

The Impact of Declining Health in a Loved One

There are some significant interpersonal changes that may come as a result of an older person's declining physical health. For families, this can include the nature of the relationship, new or additional responsibilities and the type and frequency of interactions. If the older person's declining health is impacting their ability to attend to their needs, this is often first discussed with family before assistance is delivered, either by a loved one or a paid carer. Families may be involved in arranging appointments with health professionals, co-facilitating assessments and encouraging support. Families may also be involved in supporting the older person right up to when their own health declines. This may include a wife who overnight is no longer able to provide physical support to her husband as she had a stroke and now she urgently needs care herself, as well as the responsibility on other family members to ensure that her husband receives care as well. At times care responsibilities can arise overnight, change the dynamic of relationships and be difficult to accept both physically and emotionally, particularly if delivered by complete strangers. Issues of modesty, privacy and dignity often come up.

If, on the other hand, the older person is predominately affected with cognitive changes, this may put more pressure on their adult child to monitor the older person or as described by some as 'parent the elderly parent'.

Another participant at a workshops some years ago reported: *'The move to residential care has changed our relationship as there is now a role reversal of care which can be part of the tension, as I think my mother resents the fact she cannot "mother" me as she did in the past. Also, a general lack of control of her life makes her angry and makes her feel it is my fault. It is hard to know what is the dementia and what are her true feelings.'*

Further, the impact of dementia can cause fluctuating relationship between family members, in that it can at times bring family members closer and at other times further away, as outlined by this relative: *'The condition has changed our relationship. I think for a long time, until Mum's condition worsened, it brought us closer. I had never spent so much time with her. I saw her now as vulnerable, rather than the authority figure she had always been. She needed me.'*

Tips for Others

The following tips were shared by a range of family members over the years. The advice covers strategies and information that may be useful for those who work in aged care as well as families.

Often, the first advice is about timing of the move, as illustrated by this relative: *'Don't leave the move until too late. Your parent may be in danger living alone. Mum was in danger of falls, getting lost, getting taken advantage of by others, burning the place down, as well as having poor nutrition and a lonely life. Trust the staff. Go shopping with your parent before the move for a lovely new bed cover, lamp or easy chair. Fill the room with pictures and knick-knacks they love. It is a bit like when you first left home... they went shopping with you for something lovely for your new room/home.'*

Another relative highlighted the importance of researching information beforehand: *'My advice would be to check thoroughly the aged care home you are looking at and form your own opinion and not believe everything you are told.'*

Lastly, this relative had some practical advice on what may assist: *'This move is not easy for your loved one; they will need your loving support. They will need someone that will listen to them as there will be many complaints. Sort out what are the priorities and work on that first, the other things will fall into place in time. Also keep up a good relationship with the staff and other residents as this also will help your loved one.'*

DIGGING DEEP

1. What is your experience in assisting an older person to move into an aged care facility?

2. Do you think that being stressed about moving into residential care reduces one's ability to accept the circumstance and adapt?

3. Do you feel that advice from others about the transition would help those who are going through a similar process??

CHAPTER 3

Wellbeing Factors

The vast majority of older adults experience positive ageing. This is characterised by easy adjustment to the changes in their activity levels, views on retirement and engagement in vocational, community and social activities after ceasing full-time employment. Their new routine may include paid employment in a reduced capacity, volunteer-based activities and charity work. Many cope well with emotional and physical changes faced in late life and regularly spend time with their loved ones near and far. Older people self-report greater satisfaction with life, have less concerns about finances and other pressures faced by younger generations. Positive ageing is a privilege and experience denied to many who succumb to premature death and suffering in earlier life.

However, changes in late life can be more difficult to accept if they are significant (such as a sudden deterioration in health), or cumulative, when we experience one event after another. This may include the death of a partner, changes in one's own health status or that of the loved one, or significant changes in their financial security or support network. Several retirees reported feeling 'robbed' of their retirement and the future they had planned because either they or their partner have been diagnosed with a chronic illness or dementia. Suddenly they found themselves in a new role as a care recipient versus care giver, and this was not something they expected or foresaw in their plans. The grief associated with the loss of an anticipated future can be overwhelming.

'Bob was always very active outdoors, he loved to get out and keep active. But, safety was never his priority. He somehow always managed to avoid getting into trouble until the day he fell from the roof cleaning gutters. We knew that it wasn't good when he said he couldn't move his legs. Suddenly our lives changed forever. Bob was in his early 60s when the accident happened. Over the last decade he has made some progress, however he cannot walk or even sit independently. I feel lucky, he has not had to leave home and somehow we are managing. There are hard days and frequent hospital trips, but still it is us.'

As Cheryl describes above, her husband's spinal injury had a devastating effect and changed their lives forever. She has had to learn quickly how to care for Bob, ensure he does not get pressure sores and to embrace in-home support from workers to assist Bob with activities of daily living. In the time after Bob's accident, Cheryl's parents moved into residential care. Her mother passed away about five years ago and her father is still in care. Cheryl shared the difficulties with her time management and priorities, as she feels guilty not being able to visit her father more often.

'For us, it was gradual. Denis would forget to take his shoes off or where he parked the car, to one day not remembering the name of our friends. I felt scared

and fearful of our future. I never thought we would lose our independence so early. We worked as school teachers and always had great plans of travelling the world when we retired. Suddenly we found ourselves gobsmacked with the diagnosis of dementia. I acted quickly; we sold our house, moved into a new unit and learned more about this devastating disease and how we can make the most of the time left.'

Helen is an active spokesperson as a carer and advocate for early diagnosis of dementia. She cares for her husband in their home and they have learned to embrace dementia into their retirement. Sometimes they get frustrated and Helen described the fact that it is in their face every day but that they work with it. They still spend time with their family and travel, although much closer to home and only for a few days at the time, as being in an unfamiliar environment can be unsettling for Denis.

'I was on my way to the art gallery. I remember walking down one of the main streets in Sydney when I had a fall. It was totally unexpected, sunny day, dry road and yet I just went PLUMP. They called an ambulance and I was taken to hospital. I couldn't get up. In hospital I learned that I fractured my hip. I thought ok – we will get through this. But, little did I know that it would be my last day of independence and that I would never see my unit again. My sons were informed by the doctors that my recovery would never allow me to climb the stairs to my unit and they decided that it was best for me to move into an aged care facility. I remember feeling frustrated, angry and overwhelmed.'

Betty has been living in an aged care facility for eight years. She has never gotten over that day and described sadness remembering how her life changed. She mentioned that she explored retirement villages not long before her fall, however said that she felt, 'it was for old people,' and that she did not see herself as being one of those people. Betty lost her husband when she was in her early 40s and this change brought back memories of how resilient she felt then as she had three young boys to raise – however, it also made her realise that she felt far more equipped to manage change then, than she does now in later life.

As the above examples outline, there are a number of changes which may contribute towards emotional changes and the risk of developing a mental health condition in late life. Broadly, these include changes in health status, the accumulation of grief and loss, a limited support network and the impact of isolation. The effect of sudden changes appear to have a greater impact on the individual and how they accept what has happened. This appears to be true across the lifespan – we need more time to adjust to sudden losses than gradual ones.

In addition, as we learn more about dementia and the effect it has on individuals (with little to no research on how to overcome this illness), those who are diagnosed with this condition understandably have a lot of difficulty accepting what has happened. We simply do not understand enough about it and the risk factors which appear to contribute towards diagnosis, which means many older people worry that their signs of cognitive changes may be attributed to this disease.

Raising Alarm – Whose Responsibility?

In our younger years, our emotional wellbeing is ultimately our responsibility. It is up to us to decide when we speak to a trusted individual about any changes in our emotions, and to determine when we may need to seek professional help. However, as we age and face changes in our health status, support network and potentially our environment, it must be questioned whether it is still an individual's responsibility. Particularly when older people are less likely to talk about their wellbeing.

When it comes to older people in residential care, it is important to recognise the importance of collaboration with health professionals, aged care providers and families to improve mental health outcomes. This step is essential in supporting the adjustment to a residential environment and ensuring that necessary steps are taken to promote prevention and early detection of emotional changes. Older people may not have insight into changes in their wellbeing, as they may have other barriers such as declining physical health and memory changes – but of course not everyone would have those symptoms. Individuals may be experiencing grief, loss, anxiety, depression and adjustment difficulties. Their symptoms may have been there for some time, not having been recognised by health professionals or their family. Sometimes the older person themselves may not recognise that the symptoms have been lingering for some time and may not discuss it with anyone. Unfortunately, mental health symptoms do not magically disappear or resolve themselves.

An aged care worker may have noticed that the older person is not dressed at midday, has barely touched their food and they talk about not wanting to live. All of these can be problematic and can impact care delivery and interactions between the resident and workers. Yet, the worker may think it is the responsibility of the older person rather than themselves to recognise it as a mental health condition and a symptom that needs to be escalated to health professionals. But, does this put the responsibility of mental health of older people on the workforce? Do they have the time, skills and expertise when it comes to mental health? Or, do we leave the responsibility to mental health professionals, knowing that such a small percentage works with this population and that older people are the least likely age group to seek support for their mental health? This is the challenge often faced in aged care and highlights the importance of working together.

Collaboration is crucial – between older people, their families, service providers and health professionals. Mental health becomes a shared responsibility and it is important to recognise that there are a range of ways that the older person can be supported, from practical strategies during service delivery to more formal intervention delivered by mental health professionals. Mental health conditions, just like physical health should be managed by a range of professionals. For example, with diabetes, we do not only assume that the endocrinologist would be the one to tell us to eat less sugar and be more physically active. We may hear the same advice from a range of professionals and so cannot shift the responsibility of emotional changes to mental health professionals exclusively, particularly if they are not receiving referrals for clinical work or seeing clients.

There are steps that can be taken to strengthen the resilience in older people and reduce the risk of developing a mental health condition – and it could be as simple as implementing reflective listening and encouraging socialisation.

Given the high prevalence of mental illness in older people in residential settings, as well as high suicidality in this population, it is important that we collaborate to improve mental health outcomes. This would see aged care workers knowing how to respond to a client who is emotionally distressed, having the skills to actively encourage social interaction and socialisation, knowing when to escalate concerns to management and understanding how management can work with health professionals to ensure timely intervention in support.

In practical terms, this would include:

- improved communication during care delivery
- implementing good listening skills,
- setting up residents for a successful day with good personal care habits
- reminding them of activities that are on offer that day
- providing encouragement and support to participate in onsite activities
- encouraging residents to socialise and interact with one another
- raising concerns to management of residents who are reluctant to get out of bed.

Often, the residents who are reluctant to get dressed, showered and ready, are more likely to experience emotional changes and feel a sense of isolation. The problem arises when these individuals display the same patterns of behaviour for weeks or months at a time and when these symptoms become normalised, rather than addressed early on. The longer the residents are isolated, the more difficult it can be to get them to integrate again with the environment and to make friendships with other residents or participate in activities. This could lead to an increased need for support, reduced mobility and a decline in physical health functioning. The isolated residents can be reported as being 'easy to care for', as they keep to themselves, however they are likely to require more care and support in the future as they have not been implementing resilience and skills which build on their strengths. Some of these individuals have described a loss of purpose in their lives, feeling hopeless and helpless which has stemmed from being isolated and not feeling that they belong in their environment.

Mental health in residential care needs to be a priority, to ensure better adjustment to the environment, improved outcomes for residents and a better working environment for staff. Through collaboration and inclusion of the older person in decision making around their cares and supports, this can be achieved.

Older People and Mental Health Support

Approximately 50% of the general population will seek help and support with their emotional wellbeing at some stage in their lives (Whiteford et al., 2014). They may seek advice from their GP or mental health professional, look up resources online or access a helpline. The government is spending significant funding to raise awareness about the importance of mental health across life and ensure preventative and timely support is available for those who may need it. This includes, but is not limited to, new parents, teenagers, men and people approaching retirement. However, those aged 65 and above are the least likely group to use mental health services, with less than 25% accessing support.

There are many reasons why older people are reluctant to seek support for their emotional wellbeing, including the effects of cognitive decline, experiencing several health conditions at the same time, stereotypes, misconceptions about mental health support and ageism. For older people, access to mental health has historically been controversial. Many saw it as a sign of madness and counselling sessions as check points to see if the individual 'should be locked up'. On the other hand, younger populations are more acceptive of support for mental health issues and may initiate services without those views and fears. In older generations men did not talk about their feelings, particularly those who were in major world events, such as the Great Depression, World War II and the Vietnam War. Women's role and rights have also changed, with many more women in the workforce and engaged in activities outside of home.

Both men and women in late life respond well to psychotherapy and are able to improve their wellbeing through emotional support. Older people respond to the same mental health treatment as younger people, such as cognitive behavioural therapy delivered by a mental health professional as well as enhanced lifestyle factors which contribute towards better mental health outcomes. From a therapeutic perspective, modifications required for older people include addressing sensory impairment, such as vision and hearing, and adapting the 'homework' component, tasks the older person needs to do in between counselling sessions. Lifestyle factors which have significant evidence towards enhancing wellbeing include, increased physical activity, sleep hygiene, social connection, engagement in meaningful activities and feeling included and supported in their environment. These strategies will be discussed in Part II and Part III of this book along with a practical approach to enhancing wellbeing in late life.

DIGGING DEEP

1. Do you feel that it is easy to determine if an older person is emotionally well?

2. In your experience do older people fear experiencing a decline in their health and the impact this would have on their independence?

3. What suggestion do you have for an older person to accept more help than they are currently receiving?

CHAPTER 4

Common Mental Health Conditions in Late Life

'*Oh, today he is so depressed,*' and '*she is stressed and anxious,*' are common sayings, particularly when describing older people. It is important to distinguish between personality traits, moods and mental health conditions and not apply labels to individuals who have not been formally assessed as meeting the criteria for a mental health condition. Monitoring older people, their moods and level of activities is important as well as recognising when they may require additional help and support. Monitoring and escalation of concerns can improve mental health outcomes, as older people (like the rest of the population), respond well to treatment which can improve the quality of their lives. Anxiety and depression are the two most common mental health conditions in older adults and approximately one in 20 Australians aged 65 years and over met criteria for depression and/ or an anxiety disorder (Australian Bureau of Statistics [ABS], 2008). The prevalence of depression and anxiety are much higher for those who live in residential care, with research suggesting that up to one in two residents experience symptoms of depression (National Ageing Research Institute, 2009) and that anxiety is very high, although the exact rates have not yet been formally assessed.

The rates of depression appear to rise in individuals as they age. There seems to be higher prevalence of depressive symptoms in those who are aged 85 years and over than those aged over 65 years, with studies reporting varying prevalence, ranging from 30–75% (Byrne et al., 2010; Eyers et al., 2012). The main reason for the increased rate of depression in older people is attributed to declining physical health which can impact the quality of life. When an individual has more than one health condition, such as diabetes and a heart condition, it is said that they have comorbidities. Individuals with diagnosed health conditions, such as cardiovascular, neurological, physical and endocrine conditions are at greater risk of developing mental health conditions secondary to their declining physical health. However, in some instances those individuals may have had an underlying mental health condition, such as anxiety, as a primary lifelong condition. There is no fast rule which condition comes first, but in the majority of cases it is declining physical health which affects the individual's activity levels, independence and subsequently emotional wellbeing.

According to the ABS (2007), older people with anxiety or mood disorders are the least likely of any age group to use mental health services, with approximately 23% seeking help. A similar trend was found by the American National Comorbidity Survey which indicated that older adults aged over 75 years are least likely to seek help (Fiske et al., 2009). Canadian Community Health Survey also found that seeking help decreased with age, with less than 3% of the population aged over 75 years seeking support for emotional wellbeing (Magaard et al., 2017). In the UK, the National Audit of Psychological Therapies conducted a review on all psychological services and found that older adults have the lowest rates of referrals and treatment, with less than half of the expected number (Pettit et al., 2017). There are a range of barriers for older people when it comes to their mental health, including poor detection of emotional changes by doctors who report that it can be difficult to identify symptoms and differentiate from other health conditions. Lack of patient insight, clinical presentations with short consultations focused on multiple health issues, attitudes by professionals that anxiety and depression are to be expected in older age, ageism and assumption that older people cannot learn new things and cannot participate in therapy are all additional barriers that must be overcome.

Depression

Depression is characterised with sadness, lack of interest or pleasure in otherwise enjoyable activities and persistence of symptoms for at least two weeks. Everyone experiences sadness from time to time, however, persistent feeling of low energy, low self-esteem, and low motivation is something that needs to be investigated further. Clinical depression affects emotions, physical health, cognition and behavioural aspects of life. Individuals with clinical depression often report feeling guilt, hopelessness, irritability or numbness. They may decrease participation in social activities (or withdraw from them all together), become very self-critical, believe that they have no future, experience thoughts of suicide and loss of concentration.

Depression is essentially the same disorder across our lifespan, however, some symptoms are more accentuated in older people. The symptoms of depression may include, pain and physical symptoms, memory problems, substantial weight loss, slowing down in movement, anxiety and use of different language with a reluctance to describe sadness and tearfulness. Older people are more likely to report fatigue, hopelessness and helplessness. Many older people who have depression in late life do not have a history of depression. Like anxiety, depression is a treatable mental health condition, usually treated with psychological intervention and/or medication. If left untreated it can significantly impact physical health, social connection and quality of life.

Anxiety

It is normal to feel a little anxiety or worry at times of uncertainty such as waiting for test results, being in an unfamiliar environment or being fearful of heights. Anxiety disorder occurs when an individual experiences intense physical response due to arousal of the nervous system leading to physical symptoms such as raised heartbeat and sweaty palms. These symptoms can become unescapable and interfere with wellbeing and function. Those who experience anxiety often describe an inability to cope with circumstances. They may be unable to cope with the environment, certain situations and as a result will avoid some activities.

Anxiety can be caused by several factors including heritage, biochemical imbalances, life experiences, personality, thinking style and behavioural style. Regardless of the cause, anxiety can be treated through psychological support, medication or a combination of both. Psychologists can recommend a range of non-drug approaches to reduce anxiety and improve coping strategies. Untreated anxiety can impact physical health, social connections, sleep and quality of life. If you notice early signs of anxiety in a loved one or resident, it is recommended you speak to a health professional who can provide them with coping skills to help them manage future episodes of this stress more confidently.

The term anxiety covers a wide range of conditions including generalised anxiety, panic disorder, post-traumatic stress disorder, agoraphobia and specific phobias (such as fear of spiders, snakes, driving and clowns, to name a few). The most common anxiety disorders in older people include social phobia and specific phobias. Older people tend to worry about finances, family and minor matters rather than work or interpersonal matters. Anxiety has many psychological symptoms, which include intense worry and fear, and physical symptoms, such as restlessness, tremors and sweatiness. It is thought that anxiety occurs in 5–10% of older people, with a higher prevalence in residential settings however this condition is often not screened (NARI, 2009). Anxiety is far less researched, can be situation dependant and is often easier to recognise than depression due to physical symptoms – including being fearful, agitated, experiencing sore muscles and having multiple worries. Older people with anxiety usually have a history of anxiety in their younger lives.

Adjustment Disorder

Adjustment disorder is a psychological response to stress involving marked distress and significant impairment in functioning, where the onset of symptoms is linked to a direct and identifiable stressor. Often symptoms will reduce once the individual has adjusted to the stressor. At times, responses to the stressor can be delayed and do not need to occur immediately after the stressor commences. Usually the symptoms appear within the first three months and do not last more than six months after the stressor has finished. The presentation ranges between individuals and can include depressed mood, anxiety and behavioural disturbances. In older people who live in residential care the stressor can be the move and adjustment to the new environment as well as adjustment to sudden changes in health. Like depression and anxiety, adjustment disorder is also a treatable mental health condition which can be improved through psychological support to improve coping strategies and adjustment to changes. If left untreated, adjustment disorder can impact acceptance of new circumstances, how individuals draw upon their support network, spend their time, engage in physical activities and their overall quality of life.

Grief and Loss

Grief is the natural reaction to loss, and can influence the physical, emotional, cognitive, behavioural and spiritual aspect of our lives. Grief in late life can be large or small but have an accumulative effect in response to a variety of loss-related events, such as the death of a loved one, loss of driver's licence, physical incapacity through disability, or the loss of one's home or community due to declining health or a natural disaster. Older people often experience multiple losses, such as the death of a partner, siblings, friends, declining physical health and an increased need for support. Someone who is going through grief and loss may feel lost in a maze of conflicting emotions and have a sense of losing control. To support an individual who is experiencing loss it is important to acknowledge their grief, and give them time and space to feel and remember. Be non-judgemental, allow the person to share what is on their mind, and let them know they have support. Some individuals prefer to share their stories verbally, others prefer to write them in memoirs, poems or possibly even with drawing and painting. This is discussed in more detail in Chapter 8.

Individuals cope with grief and loss in a variety of ways and there are marked difference between genders in how they prefer to cope. Women often prefer to talk more about their losses while men may prefer to be kept physically busy. Some people prefer company, while others prefer solitude. For most people, the experience of grief will dominate their emotions, thoughts and behaviours for a number of weeks or months. Most people who experience loss will not need professional help, however some seek and require professional support particularly if they are experiencing multiple setbacks including declining physical health or if their grief does not resolve. When individuals continue to experience very intense feelings associated with grief more than 12 months after a loss, this might be a sign that the individual is experiencing 'prolonged grief'.

Multiple Mental Health Conditions in Late Life

Individuals of all ages can experience more than one mental health condition at the same time. One condition can be chronic, meaning it has been present for a long period of time, and then another condition develops – for example, having a long history of anxiety and then experiencing adjustment disorder in late life. In other cases, individuals may experience the onset of both conditions around the same time, such as anxiety and depression following a health setback like a stroke. Generally, it is common to see multiple conditions on the medical files of older people or for them to disclose multiple diagnosis themselves. At times, the symptoms can overlap, which can make it difficult to disentangle which condition the symptom is attributed to – is isolation due to depression or adjustment disorder? Is reduced appetite due to an eating disorder or anxiety?

Although anxiety and depression are distinct disorders many older people may be experiencing both. Over 50% of older people with clinical depression also show evidence of comorbid anxiety (Eyers et al., 2012). Similarly, over 25% of older people with anxiety disorder show evidence of comorbid depression (Christiansen, 2001). Other mental health conditions, such as bipolar disorder (mania) is less common in old age, with prevalence at approximately 4–10% (Dols et al., 2013). Late life schizophrenia is also rare, with most cases of schizophrenia developing before the age of 45 (Dols et al., 2013). Delusional disorders in mid-life (around the age range of the 50s and 60s) is most common in females and often associated with sensory impairment, particularly hearing as well as cerebrovascular disease (Tampi et al., 2019). Paranoid type delusions are common, such as neighbours using some type of electronic device to spy through the wall, or stealing items off the washing line and from the garden. There is a high risk of comorbid medical problems and depression, with approximately 25% of clients with first presentation of psychosis after the age of 65 developing dementia within three years (Ribe et al., 2015).

Coping Through Avoidance

In psychology, avoiding certain stressors can appear to be a good measure to protect ourselves. However, avoidance can also be a negative strategy where the individual is in fact disadvantaged by their coping or escape coping behaviour. There are some behaviours specific to older people which can be detrimental to their health and wellbeing such as avoiding going out 'after dark' or alone for fear of being mugged or victimised, or avoiding exercise or other activities due to excess fear of falling or vertigo (this is particularly common in residential care, as often exercises are offered on a daily basis). Some older adults who have a sensory impairment may avoid social events due to loss of hearing, or other forms of embarrassment. Further, older people may refuse to use any type of aid to enhance functioning, such as a walker, cane or hearing aid for fear of appearing 'old', 'strange' or 'weak'. One of the common avoiding behaviours in older adults who may need more support is avoiding seeking the needed help for fear of 'becoming a burden', or losing independence and autonomy. This can become problematic as often getting the right support can easily improve the quality of life of the older person and may not be as intrusive and time-consuming as they perceive it to be. A common example in residential care is the refusal of assistance with showers due to loss of dignity and independence, yet the older person may not be able to complete the task themselves independently. There have been several instances of older people wetting the shower floor and informing staff that they have had a shower to avoid the task.

Suicidality

According to leading mental health organisation Beyond Blue, suicide is a leading cause of death in Australia. Deaths from intentional self-harm occur among males at a rate more than three times greater than that of females (ABS, 2019). The highest rates of suicide are in men aged 85 years and over (ABS, 2019). However, this trend is often not discussed in the media and many are surprised to find out suicide rates are so high in the ageing population. People aged over 65 years are more likely to have a chronic health condition present at death than their younger cohorts. Notably, cancer was present in approximately 25% of suicides and mood disorders in 26% of persons aged over 85 years (ABS, 2019). Contributing factors in old age suicide may include physical or economic dependency, mental and/or physical health problems, chronic pain, grief, loneliness, alcoholism or carer stress.

Sometimes there are warning signs of suicide that need to be considered. These include:

- a loss of interest in activities that are usually found enjoyable
- cutting back social interaction, self-care and grooming
- breaking medical regimens (for example not taking medication
- experiencing or expecting a significant personal loss (e.g. spouse)
- feeling hopeless and/or worthless (e.g. saying 'What good am I?')
- putting affairs in order, giving things away, or making changes in wills
- stockpiling medication or obtaining other lethal means.

In residential care, the risk of suicide is lower than for those who live in their own homes. While many residents may have suicidal thoughts, their access and means to end their lives is significantly lower. Medications are usually dispensed by staff, and they are closely monitored, so if they appear to not be themselves, concerns can be escalated relatively quickly to their doctors. However, a study published in the International Journal of Geriatric Psychiatry found that around 140 Australian nursing home residents took their own lives between 2000 and 2013 (Murphy et al., 2018). Researchers found that almost 70% of those who took their own life were male; nearly 80% were experiencing one or more major life stressors, such as health deterioration, 66% had a diagnosis of depression and almost 30% had found it hard adjusting to life in an aged care facility (Murphy et al., 2018). The study is the first to examine the number and patterns of suicide in Australia's nursing homes, and the largest such investigation in the world. These findings highlight the importance of understanding the risk factors associated with suicide in this population and strategies on how to improve outcomes.

DIGGING DEEP

1. Do you feel that it is easy to detect when an older person may be anxious or depressed?

2. How might grief and loss affect older people and their day-to-day lives?

3. Do you know what to do if an older person says to you that they are not coping?

Part II

Identifying Strengths

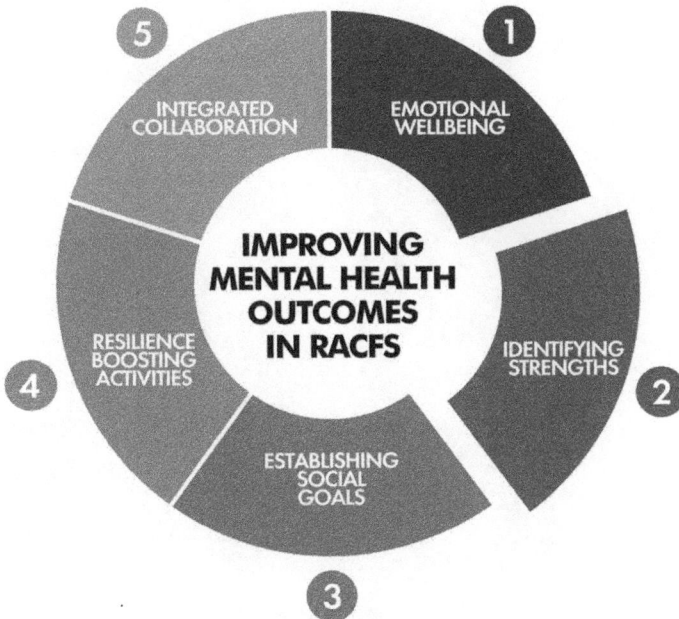

5 INTEGRATED COLLABORATION

1 EMOTIONAL WELLBEING

IMPROVING MENTAL HEALTH OUTCOMES IN RACFS

2 IDENTIFYING STRENGTHS

3 ESTABLISHING SOCIAL GOALS

4 RESILIENCE BOOSTING ACTIVITIES

CHAPTER 5

All Is
Not Lost

Betty's eyes filled with tears when she was asked if she would be participating in the wellness group discussion that morning. Betty said it was getting difficult to constantly accept help. Earlier that morning a staff member at the hostel offered to help Betty put her socks on stating, *'It is my job to help you – if I do not help you I have nothing to do'*. Putting her socks on independently was one aspect of daily care that Betty was very proud of doing herself. The staff member meant well by offering to help Betty, however in Betty's eyes it was a sign that she had lost another aspect of her independence. The morning ritual of putting on her socks and shoes meant a lot for Betty and reminded her of her strengths and ability to stand up on her own – independently.

John is a proud man who states that he rarely receives *'any care and support at all'* in an aged care facility where he has been living for the last four years. At the same time he complains of pain in his shoulders and being unable to lift his arms above shoulder height which affects his ability to wash his back. John does not welcome support from staff when it comes to showering, to the extent that he would wet the bathroom floor to trick staff into thinking he had showered just before they arrived. John would time his showers later at night when he knew fewer staff were rostered on to avoid receiving help and support. For John, maintaining his independence means that he has limited ability to wash himself – a compromise he is willing to accept.

Confidence in Late Life

For many older adults, facing health changes in late life and receiving practical support may affect their confidence and self-esteem. At times openly offering help and assuming that the individual will accept it can be determinantal to wellbeing even with the best intentions in mind. It is therefore important for help and assistance to be offered gently and mindfully, through careful wording, body language and at times the use of conversational distractions. Rather than stating, *'Let me help to shower you'*, ask the older person to share with you a pleasant memory or upcoming event, something that focuses on their strengths and current event scheduling. Opportunities to turn the relationship between care recipient and care receiver into positive interactions are endless. Delivering personal care is a delicate time when reminiscence strategies can be discussed (covered in more detail in Chapter 9) as well as topics other than the help that is being provided. Often those discussions may be the only opportunities for one on one time for the older person and can lead to deep and meaningful interactions which can uplift their mood. At the same time, it can also be rewarding for the care giver.

Delivering care and support in the mornings, provides an ideal opportunity to speak with older people about the day ahead, what activities they have planned, what the weather will be like and if there is a particular milestone that needs to be acknowledged. This approach can help to set up the older person for a successful day and put them in a good mood. Further, it can help to place a focus on their confidence, abilities and what they will achieve that day, rather than remind them of the help and supports that they require.

In our younger lives, we tend to have significantly more independence and resilience, as we not only attend to our own needs but also those of our families and children. Often, we are the nurturer and provider for our children, and also perhaps help out other family members either financially or through practical hands-on help. As we get older it can become more difficult to provide this to others, as we may need to receive help and support ourselves. John is an exception to this rule, as he attends to his daughter's lawns and helps her out in the garden as her husband is a paraplegic.

Therefore, we can help older people in late life with their confidence by discussing their stories and the experiences which have helped them through difficulties to build resilience. Older generations have wisdom and insight into current situations which can help them cope and deal with changes. We can help older people with their confidence by discussing in detail tasks they can still complete, for example managing their bills, writing shopping lists or attending to some of their cares, rather than talking about what they may not be able to complete independently any more. This approach may take some time and practice to master, however it is worth it, as building confidence in older people is important for their wellbeing and quality of life.

Identifying Strengths

If we know the older person well, it is can be easier to identify their strengths. Their strengths may not be as evident to the outside world or even the older person themselves, particularly if their physical health is declining and their independence is diminishing. The older person may have incurred changes to their psychological wellbeing, including loss in confidence and self-esteem. Subsequently, the older person may be more preoccupied about their loses and inabilities rather than recognising their strengths and abilities. While for many individuals, their strengths lie in their ability to manage activities of daily living independently, a significant portion of independence also accounts for cognitive skills, such as being able to manage finances and health issues, as well as resilience which can include having faith and practising gratitude. Psychological wellbeing is defined as a function of the qualities of the activity and the consistency with the individuals' existing structures and preferences, rather than the amount of activity engaged (Olesen & Berry, 2011). Therefore, it is important to carefully manage this process and avoid the risk of the older person feeling overwhelmed.

In essence, the task of asking the older person about their strengths is relatively simple. Strengths can be listed on a page and read out or brainstormed together. The concept behind this task is to think more broadly about their abilities, in particular, the skills which they may not easily identify themselves and how they can draw on their strengths towards developing new meaningful and engaging activities on a regular basis. Many people can become more focused on skills which they have lost due to changes in health status rather than the skills which they may have retained. The purpose of the exercise is to support the older person in identifying what they have, rather than what they have lost. To focus more on the glass half full instead of half empty approach to life and their circumstances.

Below is a list of common strengths, however, there are many more strengths an older person may have which are not listed.

- Giving and asking for support
- Setting boundaries
- Being self-aware
- Promoting acceptance
- Sitting in silence
- Having a good self-care habit
- Accepting the present moment
- Love of learning
- Forgiveness
- Giving and receiving love
- Having hope
- Being curious
- Practising gratitude
- Passion and enthusiasm
- Having faith

Strengths Based Day-to-Day Activities

Once the strengths are identified the task is not complete. It is then important to incorporate those strengths into the older person's language and day-to-day activities. This is where families and primary caregivers play a significant role. The practising aspect of any new learned behaviour is the key to mastering any skill. There are several ways in which the skill can be practised, including planning activities for the day, incorporating them into reminiscence activities as well as reminding the older person of their strengths when they are having a bad day.

When planning activities for the day, if the older person's strength is love of learning they may be interested in picking up a new hobby or attending an activity which they may not usually do, for example, art and craft activities or gardening. During an interview for my Voice of Aged Care podcast, art therapist Roxy Taylor described how some participants in her class would say they are not artists and have not painted in decades. Through exploration, many older people become more confident in their abilities to paint and create artwork, which ranged from colouring in to drawing with acrylics. It was a similar story with gardening, with some older people saying, *'I used to be a gardener,'* but once their physical health prevented them from being able to reach down to the ground and attend to their plants they had stopped. However, as horticulturist Toni Salter explained in a separate interview for the podcast, there are many ways in which gardening can be modified to allow the older person to get involved. From raised garden beds to working with smaller pots, adapting the activity allows them to participate in nurturing the garden and experience the tactile sensation and benefits of handling plants and soil.

Reminiscence through strengths is a powerful exercise which is covered in more detail in Chapter 9. Often people are fearful of reminiscing with an older person, particularly if they are bringing up topics or times when the older person was in better health or if the reminiscence involves individuals who passed away. Reminiscence can be beneficial for the older person when problem-solving and addressing any self-doubts and weaknesses, as it can remind them of their strengths and of times when they practised resilience.

Beryl is a very resilient lady who continued to live in her own house for three years after her husband passed away. Her own health was declining and she had several falls resulting in hospital admission. Beryl was aware of her declining physical health and also her loneliness living in the big house on her own. Her family were supportive but also busy with their own lives and caring responsibilities. When Beryl moved into an aged care facility she found the process daunting. She had the initial difficulty of adjusting to her environment but when we brainstormed the reasons for her admission to the facility she always brought up the decision she made when she was sitting in her garden on her own stating she no longer wanted to feel lonely. Beryl acknowledged in those moments the number of friendships she had made in the aged care home and how beneficial it has been for her health and wellbeing. She no longer felt lonely.

Experiencing health setbacks, such as pain and discomfort can affect how we feel and what we do. Older people who have had changes in medication, activity levels and possibly some unpleasant interactions with individuals can experience setbacks. Norah, for example, had decided to go for walks when her daughter visited her, but found herself in pain afterwards. Norah told me that initially she did not understand what the point of keeping active was if it only increased her pain levels. However, once she looked back through the photos taken in the lovely gardens around the facility her view changed. She acknowledged that her increased activity levels resulted in more pain and that her muscles were deconditioned. However, she was so pleased with the photographs taken with her daughter out amongst nature, she even commented, *'Look – it doesn't even look like a nursing home'.* The lesson from Norah's story highlights the power of resilience and how we can all shape our views on circumstances according to the stories we build around them. Interestingly, in Norah's case, the new outdoor adventures only encouraged her to be more active as she wanted to improve her physical health and admire the gardens more often. Her passion and enthusiasm were her strengths which helped her overcome the initial obstacle faced on her learning journey.

Case Study – Welcome Card

Dulcie was a fiercely independent lady who despite declining physical health still contributed significantly to the community of the aged care facility where she lived.

Below is a story written by Dulcie about how and why she became involved in designing welcome cards for new residents who moved into care. Through Dulcie's story you will see the resilience that beams in her storytelling and the ability to make a contribution to her environment, master how to use computers and share her knowledge with new residents. The below story was shared with me, which she typed and emailed, back in 2013. Dulcie has since passed away but the inspiration from her story is incredibly powerful.

In 2006, when I realised I would only be a burden on my friends that I worked with, as my legs were becoming rather unreliable, a friend took me to look at the aged care hostels in this area of Sydney; and in due time, I was offered respite for a month, in a residential care hostel. In the hostel someone came to welcome me, and they gave me a little hand-crafted welcome card, which I appreciated. I only stayed in respite for a week before I moved into the hostel where I am now.

What I found the hardest about the move into residential care was getting used to the new setting and finding my way around. I was shy of all the new faces of people I had never met before. I had the advantage of having a lot of my own friends, and they were so kind in visiting me. I started to learn to use a laptop, with the help of some of my friends, (by phone mostly) and have sure had to 'stick at it', but recommend it to anyone still alert enough in their mind and for diversional therapy. A knitting machine is another thing that has a similar effect as one's whole mind has to be on what one is doing! One needs good shoulders and hands for that.

So, I suggested to our care manager at that time that I could make welcome cards for new residents who moved in; and that's where it's come from! I have not stopped making cards since I started. I usually find some nice pictures on my computer and write a message and print off the card. My hands are no longer good to do the actual craft but a computer does all that for me.

I'd been asked to send in the 'history' of the welcome card and had declined before. But, now you have inspired me as I have typed this up. I do not want any formal recognition for what I do but rather a matter of interest for anyone else who may wish to explore welcome cards in the future.

Signing off
Dulcie

Case Study – Poetry

ND is a 90-year-old lady who has lived in residential aged care for the past three years. She has always shown a keen interest to participate in psychoeducation and it was during one of those sessions that I asked if she could share her views about moving into care by writing a poem. As poetry is ND's way of expressing her emotions and thoughts, she was only too happy to prepare it. What is even more impressive is that she memorised the poem and recited it to me, as well as provided a written version.

Poem written by a resident

Life Goes On
Life can change
In the blink of an eye
You ask yourself
Why me, Oh Why?

This isn't the life
I planned for myself
My dreams discarded
At the back of the shelf

But, I must keep going
I mustn't look back
They say life goes better
As you move down the track.

And, I've found for myself
It's true what they say
Life gets better
Day by Day

You can go to the movies
And have lunch with a friend
Or learn Salsa dancing
And start a new trend

You can put on your joggers
And go for a walk
And pick up the phone
And have a good talk

And don't feel sad
When you recall the past
For though people may change
The memories last

ND, 2019

DIGGING DEEP

1. How can we enhance the strengths of older people?

2. Do you have any suggestions on how to boost confidence in older people who are no longer able to live independently?

3. What strategies would help to enhance day-to-day activities for older people?

CHAPTER 6

Always
Learning

You are never too old to dream another dream or achieve a new goal.

The infamous saying above highlights the power of working towards new goals and dreams regardless of our age. Learning does not stop once we finish school, complete a course or stop working due to retirement. Learning certainly does not stop once an older person moves into an aged care facility. In fact, the adjustment to a new environment is a huge learning curve which can test an older person's resilience and neuroplasticity (the ability of the brain to change continuously throughout an individual's life), as well as short and long-term memory. Navigating a new environment can be confusing for anyone, regardless of their age, particularly for older people whose move is subsequent to declining physical health. Often families will report the sudden decline in the older person's memory once they enter residential care. In many instances it is the combination of being in an unfamiliar environment, learning new routines and the emotional impact of adjustment to the new environment which accounts for those symptoms. There are a range of strategies which can be used to assist with the move which we will discuss here in more detail.

First, let's tap into dementia. Individuals with dementia can often mask their symptoms of cognitive decline a lot easier in their own homes as opposed to being in an unfamiliar environment. This is because they know exactly where the toilet is located, how their bedroom is furnished and the layout of the entire home which can give them a sense of confidence and independence. However, once they are moved into an unfamiliar environment, families can report a sudden decline in functioning. In many instances, admission to an aged care facility can be even more problematic when the symptoms of dementia are masked well in the home environment. In those instances the adjustment to a residential environment can be more difficult, as the individual has impaired insight into their support needs and cognitive functioning. Families may report difficulties with adjustment and frequent phone calls from their loved ones requesting to go back to their home environment because they were *managing just fine at home*. This can be difficult for both the individual in care and their families. In those instances it is important to discuss changes earlier on and to be open with the individual about where they require supports, rather than doing the work quietly or without involving the older person, such as checking food in the fridge and reminding them of their appointments.

Learning is beneficial for our brain as it helps to improve our memory and our wellbeing. Learning new information and skills can be empowering and improve an individual's confidence and view of themselves. In fact, most older people who move into residential care have to do some form of learning to help them adjust to their new routine. This may include navigating around the facility, learning about meal times and activities on offer, and getting to know other residents and staff. It is almost impossible to adjust to a new environment without acquiring some new information about the layout and routine. Acknowledging the impact of the learning journey is important and allows the older person to reflect on the process and their accomplishments.

Learning is exceptionally beneficial for working memory and can reduce the impact of cognitive changes in late life. Often, older individuals have concerns about their memory in late life and the prospects of what will happen if their memory declines. Some who experience changes in their emotional wellbeing can be concerned about their memory, stating they feel it is not as good as it used to be. In those instances, if emotional changes are treated, there can be improvements in memory. On the other hand, individuals with dementia will often say their memory is good and will have little insight into their impairment. It is important to acknowledge the difference between the two and to offer support accordingly.

Types of Memory

Memory is broadly grouped into two types, short-term and long-term. Short-term memory is the capacity to hold a small amount of information in mind in an active, readily available state for a short period of time. Long-term memory, on the other hand, is broadly categorised in two distinct groups which are called declarative, also known as explicit memory, and procedural, known as implicit memory. Declarative memory reflects our ability to recall key events from our lives, such as our birthdays, how many siblings we have, the names of our parents, our children and where we have lived for majority of our lives. Many older adults can retain factual information about their background relatively well – even those who may have dementia and don't recognise their relatives can recall the names of their children and where they lived. Procedural memory, on the other hand, guides the processes we perform which involve both cognition and motor skills, such as how to bake our favourite Christmas desserts or how to ride a bike. For older adults, changes to procedural memory can be particularly difficult to accept, as they lose the skills in how to care for themselves and attend to matters and may need additional self-care strategies, such as going for long drives or attending to personal care needs and completing the task in correct order. While many may perceive showering to be a simple task, for an older person with cognitive changes this can be particularly difficult, as they need to consider when to initiate the activity, how to adjust water temperature, pick out a clean outfit, use correct toiletries and put on new clothes afterwards. This may explain why in many instances older people with memory changes can be reluctant to attend to personal care needs. It is not a matter of them not wanting to do the task, but rather, not having the skills in how to complete it. This is why offering support and encouragement is important and being skilful in how to deliver it.

There are many resources aimed for older adults which provide tips for keeping memory sharp and active. The information is useful for older people of all ages and for their families.

Dementia Australia has a number of useful and practical resources to support individuals with mild cognitive impairment and those who have a diagnosis of dementia. The following tips highlight the importance of looking after mind and body to slow down the progress of cognitive changes and associated stress (Dementia Australia, 2020).

- *Avoid harmful substances. Excessive drinking and drug abuse damages brain cells.*
- *Challenge yourself. Reading widely, keeping mentally active, and learning new skills strengthens brain connections and promotes new ones.*

- *Trust yourself more. If people feel they have control over their lives, their brain chemistry actually improves.*
- *Relax. Tension may prolong a memory loss.*
- *Make sure you get regular and adequate sleep.*
- *Eat a well-balanced diet.*
- *Pay attention. Concentrate on what you want to remember.*
- *Minimise and resist distractions.*
- *Use a notepad and carry a calendar. This may not keep your memory sharp, but does compensate for any memory lapses.*
- *Take your time.*
- *Organise belongings and use a special place for important items, e.g. car keys and glasses.*
- *Repeat names of new acquaintances in conversation.*

Cognitive Changes – Typical Ageing vs. Dementia

For many older people the fear of developing dementia is overwhelming. The persistent worry about the slightest change in functioning can induce stress and fear. Often, older people can become preoccupied with their ability to retain new information and have unrealistic expectations of being able to remember too many details. There are several ways in which symptoms of dementia can be differentiated from signs of typical ageing. Dementia Australia (2020) have identified the following 10 warning signs to look out for – if you notice any of the following symptoms in an older person be sure to make an appointment with their doctor to follow up on and they can determine if further testing is required. Some cognitive changes may be due to medication change, infections and depression and with appropriate treatment memory can be improved. However, it is important to be vigilant of the following changes and discuss them with a health professional.

1. **Memory changes that disrupt typical daily life.** Forgetting important dates or events, repeatedly asking for the same

information and not retaining the answer, relying more on reminder notes and other memory aids.

Normal ageing: Sometimes forgetting names, appointments and information relayed by health professionals but remembering them later.

2. **Challenges in planning or solving problems.** Changes in ability to work with numbers, follow a recipe, track bills or organise an outing.

    Normal ageing: Occasional mistakes when balancing accounts or omitting an ingredient when cooking (in most instances the food is still edible).

3. **Difficulty completing familiar tasks.** Trouble driving somewhere familiar, getting lost when going out for a walk, not remembering where the car is parked or the registration number of the car.

    Normal ageing: Needing to look up map ahead of travelling to a new destination, help in learning how to record a TV show or operate a mobile phone.

4. **Confusion with time or place.** Losing track of dates or seasons; forgetting where they are or how they got there.

    Normal ageing: Getting confused about the day of the week but figuring it out later, knowing the season and dressing appropriately for it.

5. **Trouble understanding visual images and spatial relationships.** Difficulty reading and comprehending sentences, impaired ability to judge distance and determine colour.

    Normal ageing: Vision changes from cataracts. Also, vision changes from other eye conditions need to be eliminated e.g. glaucoma or macular degeneration.

6. **New problems with words in speaking or writing.** Trouble following or joining a conversation, repeating themselves and not responding to non-verbal cues from others.

    Normal ageing: Sometimes having trouble finding the right word.

7. **Misplacing things and losing the ability to retrace steps.**
Putting things in unusual places (e.g. mobile phone in the
fridge or milk in the laundry), losing things, accusing others of
stealing belongings (e.g. accusing someone of pinching plants,
washing off the line or money which is not substantiated).
*Normal ageing: Occasionally misplacing things and retracing steps to
find them.*

8. **Decreased or poor judgement.** Bad moves with money and
investments (e.g. changing Will multiple times, mishandling
large amount of money), less attention to grooming and
personal care.
*Normal aging: Making a bad decision once in a while and keeping up
personal grooming consistent throughout life.*

9. **Withdrawal from vocational or social activities.** Declining
invitation to social gatherings, previously held volunteering
activities and hobbies.
Normal aging: Sometimes feeling weary of family and social obligations.

10. **Changes in mood and personality.** Becoming confused,
suspicious, depressed, fearful or anxious.
*Normal aging: Developing specific ways of doing things and becoming
irritable when a routine is disrupted.*

Every Day Matters

To assist with memory in late life it can be useful to break down the
tasks for the day and group them according to the following formula:
- useful
- active
- intellectual
- pleasurable.

These tasks do not have to be big, however, it is preferable if the older person attempts to do something new, or an activity which they have neglected for some time, such as reading (this can be as simple as reading over an old greeting card), listening to music or going for a walk. By attempting new tasks and even a different way of completing a task, such as brushing teeth with different hand, this slight change can be helpful for the brain. It helps to keep the cognitive wheels turning and improves overall memory. This task can be turned into a simple exercise completed every day whereby the older person is encouraged to think of four tasks they need to complete for the day ahead. The breakdown of the tasks can be useful in planning activities and measuring activity levels. It is not intended for the tasks to be overwhelming or too time consuming.

Often, people ask what type of activities would fall under each category. There is no rule when it comes to this as activities are unique and what is useful, active, intellectual and pleasurable to one person may not be for someone else. Below is a list of activities that some report as being helpful for them and these can certainly be modified. A card with the below formula can be found in Appendix 1.

Useful – *attending to activities of daily living such as making the bed, laundry, dispensing medication, reviewing finances, helping to deliver mail to other residents, assisting with setting up the table and attending to animals.*

Active – *going for a walk, attending exercise, stretching, gardening, dancing, taking the longer route to the room instead of the usual shortcut, social games and outings.*

Intellectual – *completing a puzzle, quiz, trivia, bingo, reading, playing a board game and having a conversation, playing a computer/iPad brain teaser game.*

Pleasurable – *spending time with friends, going for a drive, listening to music, watching a movie, spending time in a garden, painting, practising mindfulness.*

Incorporating Information Technology

In recent years the use of information technology has been embraced by many older people. Technology helps to keep individuals more independent in the community and more connected with their families. In many instances, tools and aids are used to ensure safety of the older person, such as a mobile phone, emergency alarm device and portable safety duress. It is easier to have a mobile phone nearby to answer than trying to get to a landline phone in time before it rings out. Mobile phones also provide a caller ID which enables older people to identify who is calling them before they answer the phone. Unfortunately, too many older adults in residential care get excited when their landline phone rings only to find out it is a telemarketer or a charity caller asking for a donation.

More and more older people are using mobile phones, laptops and a range of software and social media platforms on a regular basis. There has been an increased trend in the number of older people who live in residential care who FaceTime or use their Facebook profile to communicate with their families and also exchange photographs and videos. Information technology has been particularly useful for individuals with sensory impairment, such as the use of Google gadget which can answer most questions asked of Google as well as play the radio. Eleanor, who is 90 years old, found Google Play to be particularly useful due to her vision loss and isolation. She calls her gadget her best friend and asks it many questions throughout the day about the weather, current affairs and also to play her favourite talkback radio show.

Apart from mobile phones, many older people in residential care are using laptops and desktop computers. Older people in care use computers for a number of reasons, just like the rest of the society. For some, computers allow them to express their creative side, making cards (as outlined by Dulcie in Chapter 5) and typing life stories or poems. For others, it is about keeping in touch with family members, communicating with facility management on site or as a platform for learning and education. Take Janet for example, who at 82 years of age is eagerly awaiting the arrival of wi-fi at the facility where she lives, as she wants to study mental health and learn more about the human behaviour. Janet has cut out a few advertisements from the local newspaper about free online courses and she is inspired to keep learning and not let her health status or accommodation options stand in the way.

Several aged care facilities have computers on site for residents to learn how to use and to book for regular use. Most choose to bring in their laptop or an iPad when they move in as this helps to keep them connected with the family and provides entertainment. Computer use is highly encouraged for older people with declining physical health and mobility as it allows them to continue to use their working memory, enables expressionism and encourages independence despite diminishing physical health. Below is a message received from Dulcie, a former resident of an aged care facility who was always full of ideas on how to enhance the quality of lives of her fellow residents.

Hi ladies!

Got thinking last night (dangerous?) that a few of the residents were interested a couple or more years ago, in learning the basics of computing, but the office lady at the time, although she was very good on the practical aspect, the residents said she didn't have the ability to convey her knowledge.

I was wondering if it'd be worthwhile trying some computer lessons again? I don't believe I have the ability to teach, but could help with some aspects of it, maybe.

I was just Googling local lessons but it seems to be mostly written, but many free ones. I'll look some more.

Cheers
Dulcie.

DIGGING DEEP

1. Do you know of an older person who picked up a new hobby or activity late in life?

2. Why do you think older people are worried about their memory?

3. What strategies do you feel are important for an older person who wants to improve their day-to-day ability to remember?

Part III

Establishing Social Goals

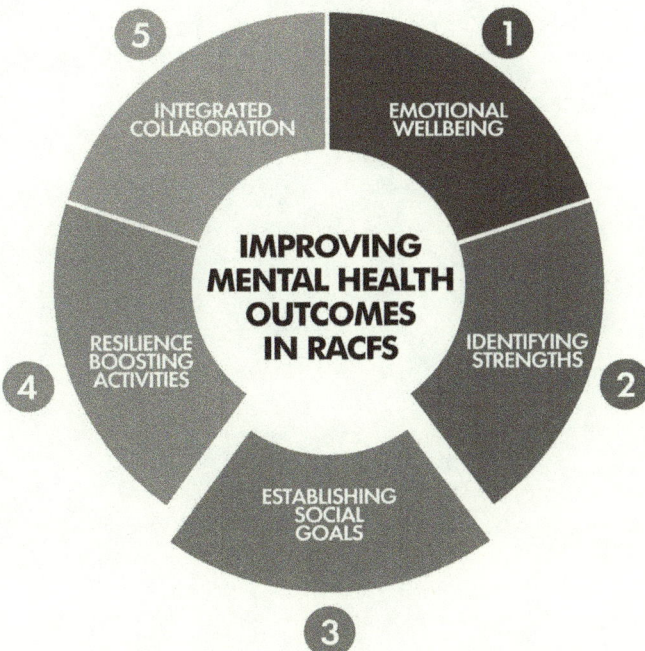

CHAPTER 7

Goal Setting

Planning and goal setting is crucial throughout life, particularly when a person experiences a setback, such as declining health in late life. At times, the importance of goals can be disregarded, with the focus placed on the losses incurred instead. In this situation, older people will often say things like, 'I used to be a gardener' or 'I used to volunteer with my arts and craft'. This suggests that they have not replaced their previous activity with another one, which eventually leads to spending a significant amount of time feeling disengaged and bored. Staying socially and mentally active despite setbacks provides a sense of accomplishment and stimulation (Stephan et al., 2008) and assists in maintaining levels of control and happiness (Tkach & Lyubomirsky, 2006).

Older people may feel disheartened about their circumstances and abilities and not see a way forward due to their setbacks. This can include dwelling on the loss of their driver's licence without exploring other options of transport, declining invitations to socialise following a death of a loved one and not wanting to go on an outing after experiencing a fall. Through careful exploration of challenges, interests and current abilities, goals can be identified and individuals supported in achieving and maintaining them. The result is that the older person experiences a new way of looking at their circumstances, and feels more confident and fulfilled. Often, there is a misconception that only the younger generations need to set goals. This could be the reason that perhaps depression, isolation and withdrawal is often normalised in the older population. There are many simple strategies that can be implemented with older people to enhance the quality of their lives and these will be discussed in detail in this chapter.

If you fail to plan, you plan to fail.

Indeed, it is important to set goals regardless of your age or health status. Goals help you plan and maintain day-to-day activities, review progress and ensure that a variety of pleasant tasks are scheduled for each and every day. Goals do not necessarily need to relate to difficult or overwhelming tasks, such as those that are popular as a new year's resolution, like wanting to lose 20 kilograms or walk 20 kilometres. Goals can be simple in nature and much more satisfying, for example, spending time in nature, gardening or listening to your favourite music. There are various approaches that can be used to set and monitor goals, including psychoeducational approach and strategies. This approach gained its name as it was developed by psychologists, but it does not necessarily mean that only psychologists should use it. The formula is simple and broken down into a step-by-step process which can be used by anyone. The beauty of its simplicity is that it is easier to master and achieve, and people feel more fulfilled if they set and attend to goals which are realistic.

In residential aged care settings, client goals are often made around care service delivery and physical health rather than the individual's emotional wellbeing and social activities. The feedback often being that facility staff feel they lack the skills to tackle the emotional wellbeing of clients and are unsure how to incorporate social goals into activity planning. The goal setting around enhancing wellbeing in older people needs to consider non-drug approaches to wellness and incorporating activities which older people find rewarding and fulfilling. Simply detecting that an older person may require counselling is insufficient and more thorough assessment needs to be carried out to identify their current interests and hobbies. Seeing a mental health professional for an hour once a week, fortnight or month will not meet all the social needs of the older person and increase their engagement in the facility. This is why a multidisciplinary and holistic approach is important, whereby the facility can demonstrate measures taken to date and liaise with various health professionals on how to enhance the quality of the older person's life. The approach may be to encourage walking (as recommended by a physiotherapist), which can be achieved by visiting the outdoor garden, minimising isolation (as recommended by a mental health professional) through encouraging attendance to small discussion groups, art therapy classes or music – the opportunities are endless.

SMART Goals

Once the importance of social goals is understood, the next step is to identify how to set and achieve them. What will be measured – satisfaction or frequency of completing the tasks? It depends on the individual and their preferences. Ideally, social goals should be more about the frequency, allowing the older person to be engaged on a day-to-day basis, rather than setting a goal down the track which may only be rewarding for a short period of time and does not increase daily engagement. The essence of social goals is to work towards achieving and maintaining them on a daily basis. Often it is the process itself in working towards the goals that people find rewarding, for example, gardening and attending to plants, rather than just eating produce, or painting rather than just admiring the finished work. The process itself can be rewarding and inspiring.

The first step when it comes to setting goals is to keep in mind the SMART goal formula. This formula summarises the essence of any goals and can be particularly useful when assisting older people who need support in setting goals. The acronym SMART stands for: Simple, Measurable, Achievable, Realistic and Timely.

Simple – goals need to be articulated in simple language with an easy to convey message. It is more appropriate to identify with the older person that they may wish to spend more time at the beach and facilitate weekly outings, rather than to plan a beachside holiday as a one-off event.

Measurable – to keep it simple, goals need to have a measure in place. Instead of having a goal of 'being happy' it may be more appropriate to identify the aim of attending social activities four times per week. That way, their activity levels can be measured in working towards the goal.

Achievable – goals should be developed in line with a person's interests, abilities and tolerances so that they can be achieved. Consideration needs to be given for older people and their mobility in how to achieve the given goal, for example, instead of stating 'spending time outdoors' it may be more appropriate to set a goal of spending 10 minutes on the balcony each day.

Realistic – refers to the importance of goals being in line with individual's circumstances. It may not be realistic for someone to have goals outside of their physical tolerance, financial circumstance or geographical location.

Timely – goals should ideally be something that the older person can achieve in the foreseeable future.

Steps to Goals

There are many ways in which older people can be supported with their social goals. The recommended approach in this book is by incorporating the SMART formula and involving the older person, health professionals and family in the process. Below is the outline for a simple four-step process. A blank copy of the template can be found in Appendix 2. It should be completed in consultation with key parties and reviewed on a regular basis – ideally monthly. This can assist the client in tracking their progress, planning daily activities and motivating them to keep active and engaged, which can significantly assist in improving their emotional wellbeing and physical health. Each party involved in supporting the older person plays an integral role towards helping them achieve their goals by providing motivation, and addressing concerns and barriers.

	Task	Notes
STEP 1 →	*Identify five enjoyable activities.*	*Enjoyable Activity 1* *Enjoyable Activity 2* *Enjoyable Activity 3* *Enjoyable Activity 4* *Enjoyable Activity 5*
STEP 2 →	*What are the client's top three strengths? (for example physical health, memory, good support network).*	*Strength 1* *Strength 2* *Strength 3*
STEP 3 →	*What are the five activities that the client is most interested in and physically able to do?*	1. 2. 3. 4. 5.

	Task	Notes
STEP 4 →	*Considering the above and current environment, what are the three activities that the client is most passionate about?*	*Activity 1* *Activity 2* *Activity 3*

Problem-Solving

One of the main challenges of goal setting is addressing problems which may arise in the process. Sometimes individuals may feel overwhelmed with barriers which prevent them from achieving their goals, and they repeatedly tell themselves and others that it is not possible for them to overcome the barriers and enjoy life. Tackling issues through a problem-solving process can help to work out solutions more proactively and address common issues. Often, individuals may only see one or two bad solutions and not explore other options and opportunities available to them in addressing the hurdles. This narrow way of thinking about the possible solutions can lead to feeling overwhelmed and avoiding solving the problem all together. This is where support and positive encouragement is necessary. A successful problem-solving process involves seven steps, which are outlined below. It is important to take the steps in a sequential order without any skipping. The task may take 15 minutes or half an hour, depending on the individual and should not be rushed or half completed. A sample problem-solving task is outlined as well to demonstrate the task.

7 Steps to Problem-Solving

Steps	Description
Step 1	Write down what the older person identifies the issue to be. Be specific and make sure you use their language in describing the issue.
Step 2	List all the possible solutions to the problem. During this process do not exclude solutions; include creative options that may seem unrealistic.
Step 3	Write down the positives and negatives of each solution.
Step 4	Help the older person rank the solutions from the worst to best.
Step 5	Assist the older person in how they could carry out the best solution and supports available.
Step 6	Put it into practice and evaluate the outcome.
Step 7	If the solution fails, choose the next best option and try again.

Problem-Solving Example 1

Pamela had several falls at home before moving into the aged care facility. She used to be active but is now worried of having another fall and avoids walking around the facility. Pamela spends most of her time in her room isolated and her physical health and wellbeing is declining. She has convinced herself that if she has another fall that she will be in a wheelchair for the rest of her life.

PROBLEM: Avoiding walking			
SOLUTIONS	**PROS**	**CONS**	**RANK**
Get facility physiotherapist to assist and review	*Learn new strategies to help with confidence*	*May have to wait a while for a session, infrequent visits, possible cost involved*	*4*
Attend exercise at the facility	*Gain deeper confidence, make new friendships*	*Time and effort*	*5*
Ask a staff member to help and supervise around the facility	*Deeper trust and confidence with staff present*	*Staff may be too busy to constantly supervise mobility*	*2*
Ask family to encourage walking	*No cost involved, more likely to have time*	*Not wanting to burden family with own needs*	*1*
Walk with another resident	*Build friendship*	*Worried about the possibility of having a fall and injuring the resident*	*3*

Calming the Mind

Stress and worry are common in everyday life, and individuals who live in residential care are not immune to it. The common topics that arise include family concerns, pending medical investigations, adjustment difficulties to the new environment, issues around interpersonal relationships with other residents and staff and at times but certainly less frequently, death and dying. Vocalising concerns about death and dying is generally not common in this population, with many accepting death as part of life and not suddenly waking up one day feeling old.

Those who have respiratory problems, such as chronic obstructive pulmonary disease, often report a fear of being out of breath. In those instances relaxation techniques can be helpful, as breathing too much can lead to hyperventilation and increase emotional distress.

Individuals who are isolated tend to have particularly high prevalence of worry, as loneliness can exacerbate feelings of hopelessness and helplessness. It is easy and tempting to say, *'Just relax, everything will be fine,'* but the reality is, this strategy often does not help to minimise the immediate stress or prevent stress from returning shortly afterwards. It is not a strategy that fixes the underlying issue or that stops the worries from arising again.

The most effective strategies are short, easy to master and sustainable. In this section we discuss several that can be easily incorporated into social goals and daily activities. The older person can practise them alone when they wake up in the morning before they receive care services, during the delivery of care services or with their loved ones. These strategies can also be laminated and enlarged if they need a reminder in how to practise them alone and prefer to do so. Instead of referring to the strategy as 'anxiety reducing' it would be more appropriate to label it as relaxation and energy boosting. If the older person is practising relaxation and their mind is calmer, they are more likely to learn new information and retain the knowledge, which can boost their confidence, memory and energy. Many older people actively look for strategies which can help them achieve exactly that.

Increasing Awareness

The first strategy in reducing stress is to increase awareness around the cause of the stress and the automatic responses made once stress has been triggered. Relaxation techniques can help individuals improve how stress is managed and there are a wide range of activities which can assist. Regularly practising relaxation helps to deal with life stressors, creates peace and calmness in daily lives and enables individuals to take better control of their emotions.

There is no right or wrong way to approach relaxation techniques and the options are truly endless, including:

- breathing strategies
- visualisation
- music
- guided meditation.

Relaxation can also extend to a wider range of activities, discussed in more detail in Chapter 8. The best approach is to try out several strategies to see which one is most appealing and then to practise it on a regular basis. Often people say they are time-poor and cannot regularly fit relaxation techniques into their daily lives. However, research has shown that even a short practice of five minutes each day can be exceptionally beneficial.

Today, there are multiple distractions vying for our attention – television, telephones, computers, family, friends and recreational activities. Somewhere along the line the art of being still and present has been lost and individuals report more frequently feeling stressed and having difficulty focusing, which leads to increased worries about memory and the impact of stress. On the other hand, meditation has been practised for centuries, focusing on the art of being still.

Many people who practice yoga are familiar with mindfulness and the benefits it brings to an individual and their wellbeing. Mindfulness is a form of meditation, which is a discipline that trains individuals how to be focused, open, curious and accepting of the present moment. It is common to experience distractions, and be hooked on unhelpful thoughts and feelings, and the purpose of mindfulness is to learn how to detach and unhook from unhelpful states without judging them. Individuals who are mindful are present in the moment, and learn how to detach from worries about the past or future. Mindfulness can help individuals learn how to respond to their present environment and the associated triggers, rather than react automatically.

Relaxing Breathing

This simple technique can be practised independently, or with the assistance of another person, such as a relative or a staff member. To begin, ask the older person to sit in a comfortable chair and place their hand on their heart while taking a few slow breaths. This allows them to observe their heart rate, as they check in with how they are feeling at that moment. For some, this will be an unfamiliar exercise. Then, ask the older person to count 10 breaths back. Encourage them to feel passive and indifferent, counting each breath slowly from 10 to 1. With each count, they should allow themselves to feel heavier and more relaxed. With each exhale, they could be encouraged to feel heavier and more relaxed. With each exhale, they could be encouraged to allow the tension to leave their body. The older person may remember this exercise straight away, but for some it can be helpful to write down the technique and provide a copy. Below is a sample text that could be used. Personalising it with their name and including an encouragement to practise it daily is also recommended.

Counting 10 breaths back

- *Sit in a comfortable chair and relax your shoulders.*
- *Allow yourself to feel passive and indifferent, counting each breath slowly from 10 to one.*
- *With each count, allow yourself to feel heavier and more relaxed.*
- *With each exhale, allow the tension to leave your body.*

Body Scan

Ask the older person to close their eyes and take 10 deep breaths. As they maintain this breathing routine, encourage them to take a moment to observe their body, noticing any tension and choosing to release it. Gently encourage them to allow their shoulders to rest away from their neck, noticing any sensations, and then bring their attention back to the breath. Next, notice their chest, their heartbeat, any sensations that emerge. If the older person becomes distracted or starts talking to you about something else, gently encourage them to bring their mind back to the breath. There is no need to be perfect with this exercise, but it is important to try and give the task a full go. Ask the older person to focus on their belly for a few breaths, asking what has emerged at that moment. Breathe into any sensation, and then release. Finally, ask the older person to explore the sensation of their legs. Often older people lose confidence when it comes to their legs and feet, with fear of falling, and bringing awareness to their legs can help to ground them. Encourage the older person to always check their feet and flooring before sitting up after the exercise is complete.

The Walking Meditation

The walking meditation is another simple task that can easily be completed with older people individually, or in a small group. The goal of this exercise is for the older person to become aware of their walking, breath and thoughts. It is important to try and schedule this activity when there are less distractions around, such as loud noises, crowds and extreme weather (in particular heat). Ask the older person to focus on their feet on the ground, and encourage them to start taking slow steps and notice their posture. Are they feeling relaxed or tense? Encourage them to notice their legs and the energy within them as they take steps. How is their body? Is there any tension? They may tense, then release. Encourage the older person to mindfully take steps, and to be as present as possible in the activity. If their mind wanders, simply ask them to bring it back to the present moment. They may label the thoughts as 'thinking' or 'planning'.

Gratitude

It is easy to focus on the losses and disappointments in life. Often when talking about accomplishments and gratitude people tend to generalise and say they are grateful for their family, roof over their head or financial security. However, being mindful in more detail about gratitude allows individuals to dig deeper into what occurs around them on a daily basis and discover simple pleasures which they enjoy. This task is again very simple and can be completed in five minutes. The older person can choose to write down what they are thankful for, or just take a few minutes to identify three positive things that happened for them that day. They can start with three items and increase in time. As they complete this exercise, encourage them to notice their breathing and any accompanying sensations in their body.

Grounding

This is another simple exercise, but it requires a bit more time than the above tasks. It teaches the older person how to bring themselves back to the present moment anywhere and anytime using their five senses to connect with the here and now. First, ask them to identify five things they can see (e.g. one specific colour in the room, one single object or the light reflecting around you). Next, focus on four things they can hear (this can be problematic for some with hearing impairment and can be omitted), then move on to identify three things they can touch, then two items they can smell and one final thing they can taste. Each time the mind gets distracted, encourage them to bring their attention back to the here and now.

As a suggestion, it is recommended to complete the task in the following abbreviated version before moving on to the full version.

What are three things you can see?
What are two things you can hear?
What is one thing you can touch?

DIGGING DEEP

1. What aspect of SMART goals do you feel older people struggle with the most?

2. Do you have any suggestions on how older people who are stressed may be able to embed relaxation into their daily lives?

3. Do you regularly engage in relaxation activities yourself (i.e. sleep is not relaxation!)?

Part IV

Resilience Boosting Activities

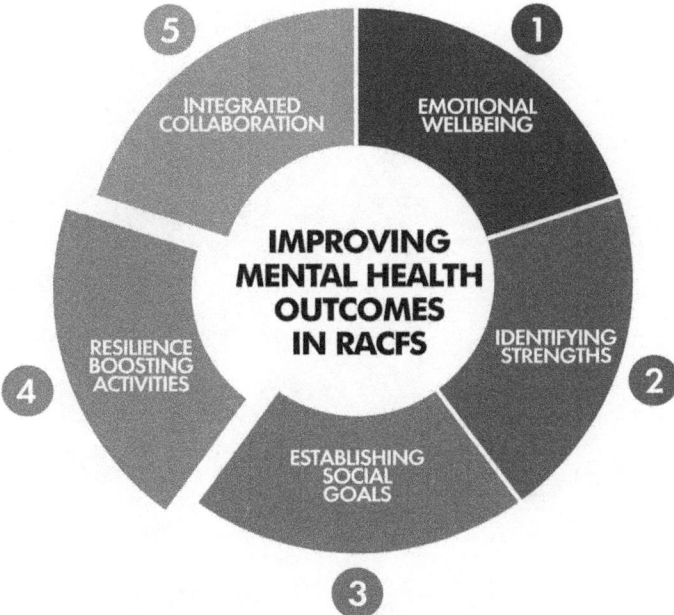

INTEGRATED COLLABORATION

EMOTIONAL WELLBEING

IMPROVING MENTAL HEALTH OUTCOMES IN RACFS

IDENTIFYING STRENGTHS

RESILIENCE BOOSTING ACTIVITIES

ESTABLISHING SOCIAL GOALS

CHAPTER 8

Onsite
Activities

Psychosocial strategies include any interventions that emphasise psychological or social approaches, rather than biological intervention such as medication. Unfortunately, the effectiveness of psychosocial strategies is often not well understood, predominately because until recently they have not been used and assessed as extensively as biological interventions. There has been a big shift in the activities offered onsite in residential settings, with the focus on delivering activities that are in line with the interests of older people as well as new innovation incorporating information technology and animals. The main issue for a number of organisations appears to be sustainability – the ability to run services on an ongoing basis. Sometimes staff require additional skills to offer these strategies, other times they need to think more broadly about how they approach their roles and incorporate feedback from their clients into service delivery. They may run regular surveys and open forums to better understand what type of services appeal to the clients and to investigate low attendance in some of the activities. Encouragingly, there is a growing awareness around offering a wide range of interests and hobbies to meet the needs of all (within budgets of course).

There is a common misconception that activities in an aged care facility are the same as entertainment, and many facilities organise singers, dancers and performers. While many older people enjoy music, as outlined below, it is important to recognise that it is not for everyone. Just like putting on a DVD and continually playing a musical is not in everyone's interest. Here, a range of psychosocial strategies will be discussed and reviewed, with steps outlining how they can be incorporated into facilities. The full list of strategies can be found in Appendix 3.

Spending Time Outdoors

Breathing in fresh air and spending time outdoors can lead to a number of general advantages for overall health and wellness. The open air provides many possibilities for individuals of all ages to be more physically active and alert than being indoors. When spending time outside, individuals learn to respond to the elements of the nature (sun on the face, wind in the hair) and to be mindful of the surrounding greenery. This awareness can help enhance mental health and reduce stress. Spending time outdoors with an older person who lives in an aged care facility is beneficial for their wellbeing and alertness and is something that should be encouraged on a regular basis, particularly if the person is constantly exposed to air-conditioned and indoor air. Regardless of the older person's mobility, time outdoors can be facilitated with the help of aids. Activities can be arranged outdoors, family visits as well as some time alone or with other residents. Older people have a lifetime of experience spending time outdoors and this can help with their memory, as well as encourage reminiscence and improving alertness.

Being in direct sunlight is the human body's main source of Vitamin D, however people tend to get occupied with the negative effects of spending too much time in the sun, such as skin cancer and heat stroke. Often it is forgotten that even spending a few minutes can be beneficial. Research has shown that as little as 10 minutes of sun exposure a day can help increase a person's levels of Vitamin D, which has been known to help fight off osteoporosis, cancer and depression (Kerr et al., 2012). Deficiency in Vitamin D is common in older people and many take medication to boost their levels. Timing of an outdoor activity is important – some may feel more comfortable being outdoors early in the morning before the day gets hot, some may find it rewarding soaking up some sunshine on their skin in the middle of the day, while others may enjoy being in the afternoon sun or watching the sun set. Spending time in the sun can assist with healing and speed up recovery from an illness or injury. Studies show that those exposed to more natural light have quicker recoveries and experience less pain than those exposed to artificial light (e.g. Kerr et al., 2012). This can be particularly useful for older people who have recently had an illness, have a reduced immune system or those who have recently undergone surgery.

When individuals are outdoors, they are more likely to engage in physical activities than when they are inside. For example, being outside can encourage you to go for a walk, take up gardening, water plants and many other recreational activities to maintain optimal physical health. Older people enjoy being kept involved and included, especially when they feel they are contributing and participating in meaningful activities. Group activities such as gardening, or even setting up a seated activity or exercise outdoors can be more beneficial for physical and emotional health than if the same activity was offered indoors.

Activities do not necessarily need to be long in duration, even thirty minutes each day mid-morning would be beneficial and engaging.

One of the common complaints made by older people in residential setting is their boredom or lack of engagement in meaningful activities. For many, having their laundry and cleaning taken care of reduces the number of tasks they complete themselves. Although it may initially sound great not having to do any housework, in the long run it can lead to an increased sense of isolation, and a lack of engagement and purpose. Going outside can improve our cognitive engagement and get our brain moving and processing. Even if an older person simply sits outside or takes a short stroll, independently, with a walker or in a wheelchair, the sensory stimulation provided by nature can eliminate boredom and improve overall engagement.

Older people in residential care often report feeling lonely and isolated. They may not be familiar with their neighbours in the facility, or had an opportunity to meet with others with whom they may be sharing interests. This can mean there are a group of older people sitting alone in their room in the same facility. An outdoor space allows older people more opportunities to socialise. Spending time with other people can boost self-esteem and positivity, and keep them from feeling lonely and out of touch. A number of psychological studies have linked time spent out in fresh air and sunshine to a greater sense of vitality. Not only does being outside give you more energy throughout the day, but vitality also helps our bodies become more resilient to physical illness.

Finally, time outdoors can lead to a greater feeling of happiness. Humans have a natural connection to living things, such as flowers, greenery and wildlife. When we are out in nature, it is easy to feel like we belong in our environment and foster a sunny disposition. This time can also help older people accept the change in their health and environment, which can lead to more open and frank discussions than those held indoors. Nature can foster a safe environment for some conversations and encourage older people to recall happier memories in their lives.

Music and Arts

Music and arts are embraced in a number of facilities. This includes listening to musical recordings, live performances as well as background music played in dementia wards. Arts is a broad term, which includes craft activities, knitting and painting. To understand how music and arts can benefit those in an aged care facility, I interviewed an art therapist and a music therapist to find out what is involved in their line of work and how they structure their visits. Below is an outline of each service delivery as well as its effectiveness in addressing the emotional needs of older people in residential care.

Art Therapy

Art therapy is a creative intervention developed to help individuals creatively express their emotions through art. It is believed to be beneficial to all, regardless of their health status and talent for art. Art therapy has been recognised as having a positive impact on wellbeing, anxiety and depression in older people. However, more research is required to determine its effectiveness in a larger sample. While many residential aged care facilities may have arts and craft on offer as an activity not as many engage a qualified art therapist who works with clients to create original pieces of art.

Art therapists visit aged care facilities (some are even employed by them) and work with individuals to determine their strengths and abilities in visually expressing themselves. An art therapist may have a room full of people and they may all use different mediums while working alongside each other to create their work.

As art therapist Roxy Taylor describes, in an interview for the Voice of Aged Care podcast (2019): *'I can have a group, there can be seven people ranging in different needs, different levels of dementia but I try to have everyone working on something that is important to them. So, what ends up happening is that the artworks end up kind of speaking for themselves.'*

For some, talking about their emotions can be difficult and art can help them express how they feel in a creative way. Art therapy session foster a safe environment where the individual can relax and enjoy an activity which takes the focus away from their worries and pain. In the end, the artwork they produce can be shared with their loved ones with digital reproduction into cards, smaller prints or original works.

Case Study – Client with complex mental health needs

Barbara has a history of complex mental health issues. Her room was full of art, framed photographs of flowers, pets and some paintings. She proudly said that she used to paint, however, was worried about resuming painting, as she thought that other residents in the facility may ask her why she has not been painting for a while. A psychologist worked closely with the art therapist and Barbara. Through problem-solving techniques, Barbara identified the best solution from a range of options. This included showing up early for the class and getting herself set up, so that when others came into the room she would already be present. This worked well for her and she continues to paint to this day. The art therapist also visits her before the class to check up on her and encourage attendance. Art therapy has been very effective for Barbara and has helped to reduce her anxiety and isolation.

Music therapy

A music therapist uses music to help someone deal with stress, anxiety and/or depression to overcome their problems and enhance wellbeing and quality of life. Music appears to affect the brain systems that control emotions. There is significant evidence on the effectiveness of music and singing with older people, particularly in improving wellbeing, and reducing symptoms of depression and anxiety.

Music therapists plan sessions ahead of their visit, however, they often need to adjust the session to match the mood of the residents. A music therapist's role is not to deliver entertainment and make everyone happy and jolly, but rather to focus on individuals and check in with them and how they are feeling on the day. Often, music therapists will play some popular songs which resonate with older people but also allow the elderly to engage more broadly in the session by playing the instruments and creating their own music. Music therapists work on both an individual and group basis. Some are employed by facilities, whilst others come as visiting contractors.

There is a huge difference between having a qualified music therapist on site at an aged care facility versus listening to a recording or having a live concert. Music therapists are involved more personally with clients and can adjust the type and tone of music to match the mood of clients and to connect better with them. When I interviewed music therapist Johanna Haire, for the Voice of Aged Care podcast, she beautifully summarised the role of music therapist:

'I'm not going to go in there and be all jolly and try to wake everyone up. That's not what I do. I will go in there and I will match the mood, so I'll start off gently and then slowly try and warm up the room and address individual people to see what they need. So not everyone wants to be jollied along or cheered up. Some people are happy to come along with me, others prefer to be left to sleep in their chair. And generally, but not always, at the end of the session after some singing or some recorded music, maybe some dancing or some instrument

playing, generally, I will find that the mood has lifted and people are brighter, and happier, I would say.'

Physical Activity

Therapeutic Gardening

Gardening is the practice of growing and cultivating plants and has been shown to help with promoting wellbeing in older people, as well as help to reduce symptoms of depression. At present there is no significant evidence to suggest that it can assist with anxiety, however, in my podcast interview with horticulturalist Toni Salter, she discusses how in her experience nature-assisted therapy has been helpful in reducing stress, including her own, Many people turn to gardening as a form of relaxation and nurturing, as it gives them satisfaction to see their efforts when the garden blooms.

Many older adults would use the term, *'I used to be a gardener,'* in an aged care facility, however not as many would engage in gardening on site. In my experience, some embraced gardening after stating they felt bored with the craft activities offered on site. Aged care facilities often have raised garden beds, but they are not necessarily used, particularly in dementia wards. This has created an opportunity for those who like gardening, to engage (through self-initiation) in this rewarding activity with the assistance of their friends and family, who can organise a trip to the local nursery to source seedlings and seeds.

Aged care facilities can easily incorporate gardening into their weekly program. As suggested by Toni Salter, activities may be as simple as smelling some herbs, or be more involved such as spending time in the garden. Protective gear is particularly important for older people, such as protection of skin from soil as well as sun exposure. If an individual is unable to physically engage in gardening, they may still be able to observe the activity which they may find rewarding. Further, there seems to be a great level of satisfaction in watering the garden and often a couple of residents seem to be particularly keen to assume this responsibility and this task in itself is not only beneficial for the garden, but it can also assist with increased physical activity.

Exercise

The vast majority of older people dislike the word exercise, and instead prefer to use words such as walking and keeping active. Physical activity, which includes a range of activities aimed at improving cardiovascular functioning, is very beneficial for emotional wellbeing, and research shows it is helpful in reducing the symptoms of depression and anxiety (Eyers et al., 2012) as well as enhance cognitive functioning and reduce the risk of dementia (Farrow & Ellis, 2013). Exercise in aged care is often facilitated by lifestyle employees, however physiotherapists and other allied health professionals may also be involved. In my own experience, most exercises are performed seated, to reduce the risk of falls in clients and provide extra support. Exercise classes usually last for about 30–45 minutes. They may include stretch bands, balls, small dumbbells and balloons. The aim of the session is to increase the use of muscles and also to boost socialisation. Many older people may have been active previously through walking groups and dancing, however once in residential care their activity levels may have reduced. The risk of falls is particularly great for those who are not physically active and who do not engage in exercise, however motivation to attend exercise can be an issue.

Many gyms reward their members for reaching certain milestones, such as three month, six month or annual memberships. This incentive can be incorporated into the aged care context whereby the residents are recognised for the effort put into exercise. A simple attendance certificate can boost self-esteem and encourage an individual to keep doing what they are doing. A sample certificate is provided in Appendix 4. This strategy may assist in boosting participation numbers in exercise and encourage those who do not attend regularly to attend more often.

Recognition can be made for attending the first 10 sessions, or more significant milestones such as 100 sessions.

Late in 2019, I interviewed Michelle Harrison and Michael Thomas for the Voice of Aged Care podcast. Michelle and Mike own a business called Love to Live Angels. They run group classes in aged care facilities which last about 45 minutes. The classes are filled with exercise, dance moves and laughter and they have made hundreds of older people feel good. Michelle shared how one of her clients did not want to go on an outing with their family, as they did not want to miss the class.

Social Activity

Pet Therapy

Animal and pet therapy is a group of treatments where animals are used by a trained mental health professional. Animals can also be used in less structured ways to provide companionship in residential care settings. Interaction with animals has been shown to improve wellbeing in older people and is particularly beneficial for individuals who experience symptoms of depression.

The human-animal bond is special and has been researched for decades. In particular, it is believed that there is a special kinship between dogs and people of all ages. Attention from a dog can brighten your day, make you feel loved and, has been scientifically proven to improve overall health and wellbeing (Cherniack & Cherniack, 2014). Introducing animals in a therapeutic way with those who are in poor health is not a new phenomenon. Animals help boost interaction and companionship in hospital, rehabilitation and residential care settings. In residential settings engagement ranges from permanent onsite animals to scheduled visits with a volunteer-based organisation. The frequency and level of animal engagement varies greatly between facilities and depends on the animal, availability of individuals (and animals!), profile of residents, their interests as well as geographical location. In some metropolitan areas it may be easier to facilitate visits than in regional and rural areas. Whereas, regional and rural areas may have more exposure to farm animals and onsite pets than a metropolitan area.

Interacting with animals has physiological and psychological benefits for humans. Physiologically, the interaction includes an increased level of physical activity, ranging from reaching out to pat an animal to getting out and about with an animal, such as taking a dog for a walk or attending to an animal's feeding routine. We have known for a long time the benefits of mobility dogs for those with vision impairment, however in recent years there has been an increase in the use of dogs for emotional wellbeing. Psychologically, it is believed that interaction with animals boosts confidence and fosters an increased sense of acceptance and empathy.

Many older people have grown up with pets and through scheduled volunteer visits are able to again connect with animals despite their declining physical health and their surroundings in an aged care environments. The interaction with animals can help to foster a safe space to reminisce about the past and create a safe and nurturing environment. It is not uncommon to observe a warm interaction between animals and residents of aged care facilities who are otherwise quiet and not engaged in other activities. A past client developed such a warm bond with a resident cat of an aged care hostel that she took it as her responsibility to feed the cat and would often save some of her own meals, particularly prawns and chicken, to feed the cat the best possible food. Sadly, the cat died only few days after this lady passed away.

Through volunteer organisations visits can be facilitated, most commonly with dogs, but visiting animal farms are also possible. Some facilities have resident pets on site, most commonly birds and fish, as they do not require a significant amount of time to care for. Nowadays, there is an increased awareness about the risks and safety of having animals on site and ensuring that the environment can facilitate an animal on a full-time basis. For example, a Sydney-based facility obtained a dog, but when management changed it became a problem, as the manager used to take the dog home with her. After a few foster homes and many consultations with residents the dog found a forever home with another staff member and continues to be on site most days, much to the delight of the residents.

In recent years there has been an increase in the number of dogs that visit nursing homes. Most often the dogs are either owned by the residents, their relatives or organised through a volunteer scheme with scheduled visits. In late 2019, during my podcast interview with a volunteer from an Australian-based society which facilitates interactions with dogs, she shared her experience and what it takes to become a volunteer. She also explained the requirement for the dog to pass tests to determine if their temper, attitude and health is suitable for visiting an aged care facility. During the interview, the volunteer also shared the amazing level of insight of her golden retriever who has been visiting aged care facilities for many years. This dog recognises when someone has a reduced mobility and knows how to approach them as she gets closer. She can also recognise if someone has had a stroke and will automatically get closer to the side of the body which is unaffected.

'Jazzy, the therapy dog knows, and I don't know how she knows, but she instinctively goes up to and puts her head near a hand that works. So, there might be a stroke victim that can only move one arm and she knows which arm to go to. I don't know how she does it but it's pretty much 100% of the time she'll pick the right arm to go to.'

Recognising that animals share a special bond with humans is important – even more so in an aged care environment which is characterised with declining physical health and barriers to recovery.

Men's Group

Often men in aged care facilities can be isolated. They may struggle to relate to the activities on offer on site and find that they are often more suitable for females. Men's group is a semi-structured session, facilitated by a volunteer or a facility employee, which allows men to discuss their issues and concerns in a supportive environment. There is significant research that suggests Men's Sheds are beneficial for men, to help them socialise and undertake enjoyable and meaningful activities. However, once the men experience health decline, they may no longer be able to physically participate in such activities. Men's group is suitable for all men in aged care facilities regardless of their health status. They discuss a range of topics and are gently guided by a facilitator in how to turn their negative experiences into strengths and form friendships with other residents.

A highly experienced men's group facilitator, Bob Creelman, shared his experience in facilitating men's group with me in a podcast interview for the Voice of Aged Care. Bob has been working with men's group in an aged care facility for over a decade. In the interview, Bob shared the importance of discussing grief and loss with men, particularly if their spouse has passed away and the importance for men to have an opportunity to do this with other men. Bob also mentioned how important it is to discuss the death of members in the group, which allows the process of natural grief and insight into the environment and surroundings. Death of other residents is often not discussed in aged care facilities and this is something that Bob feels strongly about.

'It became, for them, a type of a refuge in many ways. I have some of them say to me, "I just love this Men's Group. It is just so good". One fellow we had had to move from one facility to another and he found that very difficult. But the link that enabled him to cross was his attendance at the men's group, because he felt he was going to a strange area but the men's group was there so it wasn't so strange.'

Reflection

Reflection includes activities such as reminiscence, prayer and spiritual counselling. Reminiscence is such an important intervention to boost wellbeing in older people that it has been addressed separately in Chapter 9. Prayer and spiritual counselling, on the other hand, are briefly reviewed here, as their effectiveness for emotional wellbeing and mental health is not as well researched. Some emerging research indicates that this intervention is effective for general wellbeing in late life and that it can help to reduce social isolation and depression.

Prayer is the act or practice of praying to God, another deity or an object of worship. A number of aged care facilities employ chaplains and pastoral practitioners who form a part of a chaplaincy team. In some facilities services are formally structured with weekly one-hour chapel sessions, while in others, sessions are far less frequent and the work is usually conducted individually with residents. One of the fascinating aspects about prayer and spiritual counselling is that many people continue to be able to engage in this reflection activity despite the changes in their health. Many older people have told me that they start and finish the day with a prayer and how it helps them process the challenges of the day ahead, as well as reflect on what occurred in the day. I have also had clients return to their rooms after lunch for some quiet time and prayer, as they find that they cannot practice this being surrounded by other people during the day. They reported that prayer alone allowed them time to reflect on their day and put some thoughts together about their blessings, including their families and relatives.

Prayer is thought to give people a sense of comfort, ease and protection, therefore decreasing irrational fear and anxiety. Many people who engage in regular prayer report positive benefits on how it helps to calm their mind and accept changes in late life, including grief and loss.

The chaplaincy team in aged care facilities provides support to residents, in particular if they are approaching the end of their life and need additional pastoral support. Support is also offered to families and relatives of residents, as well as those who have been diagnosed with a chronic health condition, to help them accept and come to terms with changes in their lives.

Meditation and Relaxation

There are many benefits of meditation and relaxation for individuals and their wellbeing, in particular those experiencing anxiety and depression. There are a variety of relaxation techniques that can be practised by staff using simple aids such as relaxation recordings, which can be downloaded from internet. Relaxation strategies can be incorporated into exercise routines and other activities in the last 15 minutes of the session. Some facilities may run a separate relaxation session with the residents in a seated position.

Relaxation strategies help to ground individuals and focus their breathing and mind on the present moment, instead of fast, fleeting thoughts about the future and obstacles ahead, or dwelling on their past. Relaxation strategies are particularly beneficial for individuals who may be experiencing symptoms of anxiety and are not sure how to reduce those symptoms independently. Some report that meditation strategies appear complex and ambiguous and they are unsure how beneficial they are for them, if at all. This illustrates how important it is for those facilitating these strategies to deliver them in a simple way and with confidence, allowing older people to embrace the exercise and help them master the task to practise later on their own.

There are several easy strategies that can be used, such as meditation that focuses breath on our bodies, also known as a 'body scan', and breathing to slow down and calm the racing thoughts that are rushing through our heads. Some of those strategies and steps have been outlined in Chapter 7.

Many relaxation techniques focus on our breathing, allowing us to reflect on how quickly we breathe in and out. These techniques can help older people, particularly those who experience anxiety, to slow down their breathing and in turn calm their thoughts. The exercises are easy to learn, however require practice to master them – not because they are complex, but because they are so simple and that some people brush them and their benefits off. Therefore, it is particularly important to be encouraging the older person to practise them on a regular basis.

In another interview for the Voice of Aged Care podcast, I spoke with Liz Kraeftt, a qualified yoga instructor, who shared the importance of slowing the breath. In the interview, Liz discusses the techniques which her students embrace and how she has a growing number of older people who attend the sessions wanting to improve their relaxation strategies in late life. Liz discusses the importance of regular practice, either alone or in a class setting, to master the skill and to fit it into their daily schedule. Sometimes we can brush off techniques for the perception that they are too easy and not as important, however they can be the tasks that illustrate exactly what we need at a given point of time.

Liz discusses the concept of ageing with yoga and how different poses can be improvised if the older person has mobility issues: *'What I found is our regular students who have aged whilst they have been practising yoga have not got many mobility issues because they have been practising for a long time. However, we are always getting people start who are new to the practice and mobility can be a problem. If you find it a struggle to get down to the floor (and get up again), what we do is modify things by using chairs. And if people cannot get to the floor, the chair is a very useful prop and everything can be done from the chair including a propped seated position for when you move into some relaxation.'*

DIGGING DEEP

1. What onsite activity do you feel is the easiest to maintain in an aged care facility?

2. Why do you feel that older people may be reluctant to exercise?

3. Do you think that it is beneficial to organise activities specific for men in residential aged care?

CHAPTER 9

Sharing
Memories

Everyone engages in reminiscence from time to time without even consciously realising it. Reminiscence includes thinking about and sharing memories which are special and important to an individual. This may include memories of our favourite holidays, childhood memories without technology or getting up to mischief and special memories with people who are no longer with us. Reminiscence is a powerful psychosocial technique, which covers a wide range of techniques that involve describing past experiences that are personally significant. Often individuals choose to reminisce on their own, without discussing their thoughts and memories with others. Otherwise, reminiscence is done in pairs, or small groups. Reminiscence is a powerful way to enhance the quality of interactions, and for older people in particular, to improve their memory.

Many would have fond memories of their grandparents telling them stories from their youth time and time again, even though the older person may not have any cognitive impairment. Reminiscence is not about factual storytelling, it is more about how the individual perceived the event and the importance it has for them. The purpose of the reminiscence is not to drill down to the factual information, unless of course you are before the court and need to produce evidence. Interestingly, often even in those situations, eyewitness recall greatly differs from person to person.

Broadly, reminiscence covers three types of interventions which include: simple reminiscence, life review and life review therapy. Reminiscence is powerful regardless which format it is used in, whether simple or more formally in therapy. Evidence suggests that it is the frequency of reminiscence and how it is incorporated into daily living that makes it particularly beneficial for older adults who may be experiencing declining physical health and changes in their environment (Gibson, 2011). Reminiscence has been found to be beneficial for individuals who have sensory impairment, depression, come from culturally and linguistically diverse backgrounds and those who are terminally ill or bereaved.

Recently, an elderly gentleman in an aged care facility was identified as requiring psychological support due to his isolation. The client had not been at the facility for a long time, perhaps a few months, but staff noticed he was not mixing with other residents and spent most of his time in bed sleeping. He was socially isolated, with only couple of visitors and no family contact and his hearing was quite impaired. Several attempts were made to review this gentleman and each time he appeared to be asleep. Finally, staff asked for assistance in arranging a psychological review and ensuring the time was suitable for the resident. After some initial adjustment, including finding the hearing aids and establishing rapport the next hour was spent listening to this gentleman's storytelling about his past and his decision to disengage from the nursing home environment and instead close his eyes and reminisce about his past travels abroad. This was his coping strategy and one he used on a regular basis to help him cope with adjustment. His hearing was not as impaired as initially described, he did not seem to have difficulty hearing with the hearing aids, and his need to share his rich stories from his travel were very important to him. He spoke of times when he needed to show resilience, strength and determination – all the skills required to help with his new environment and isolation. He welcomed the psychologist to see him again, and at the conclusion of the session he had a big smile on his face and he was wide awake.

While there are many benefits to reminiscence, there are also barriers. Often individuals state that they simply do not have the time, skills or confidence to engage in reminiscence with older people. Sometimes, individuals are afraid that reminiscing can bring up negative emotions in older people, or evoke responses for which they may not know how to respond. However, if we do not start engaging in reminiscence we will find it more difficult to get to know older people, their needs and preferences. By practising reminiscence and giving it a go a lot of those barriers can be overcome.

Skills Required

Often, people think they are not 'qualified or experienced' to use reminiscence in their role. You do not need to have tertiary qualifications to engage in reminiscence. There are two main requirements for reminiscence: time and good listening skills. Even engaging in some simple reminiscence for a few minutes is effective and can be done while delivering daily activities, such as attending to personal care or a walk. As for active listening, this requires the skill of being able to listen to hear, not necessarily respond. Allow the person to share their knowledge and experiences without judgement and pressure.

Other skills required for reminiscence include:

- empathising – sharing another's world without losing hold of your own
- attending – being available to people
- relating sensitively – not being a bull in a china shop
- being non-judgemental – accepting people as they are
- not being frightened by the expression of painful emotions
- being able to enjoy reminiscing and be interested in the past
- being disciplined, but willing to share personal stories
- being able to reflect upon, accept and offer criticism of the work done.

Like many skills, reminiscence skills grow with experience. The more you engage in it, the better you will get at it. Your confidence will grow and eventually you will feel comfortable in initiating reminiscence with older adults.

Incorporating Reminiscence with Older People

There are four key aspects to incorporating reminiscence with older people which are beneficial. These are – talking, reflecting, life review and production of a tangible record. Talking encourages the older person to share their stories without judgement or pressure and for the listener to actively listen, help the older person reflect, and formulate some of the stories into a structure. This will assist with the second stage known as life review, which reviews some of the key milestones achieved. Encourage the older person (and their families) to retain cherished possessions and memorabilia, as they provide continuity, familiarity, comfort and pleasure in the present. This may include photographs, copies of achievements or souvenirs from favourite holidays. Having these items readily available and on display can trigger happy memories for older people on a regular basis and assist with frequent reminiscence.

There are three broad approaches to reminiscence which include simple reminiscence, life review and life review therapy. Each approach is outlined below.

Simple Reminiscence

Simple reminiscence, as the term suggests, is used often and by many individuals. In aged care in particular, it may include some conversations starters such as looking at the picture on the wall and asking, *'Who are the people in this photo?'* with the anticipation that it will open up a conversation with the older person. Sometimes there are no prompts with simple reminiscence, it can be more the case of opening a conversation and asking the older person about a certain event in their past. There is no structure to how the questions are posed and it does not consist of autobiographical storytelling. The older person is simply describing events from their past with little cue or direction from the other person. Even in this form, reminiscence is beneficial, as the storyteller shares their experiences and interpretation of events.

Life Review

Life review is a structured form of reminiscence and requires more time and thought into questions ahead of the session. With life review, individuals are helped to re-evaluate their lives and make use of coping strategies which they acquired over the years. This intervention assists individuals to resolve conflicts from their past and to see their lives in balance – increasing feelings of gratitude and reducing feelings of despair. With life review, the focus is on systematically reviewing different life stages and how the individual coped with those transitions, including:

- childhood friendships
- education and schooling
- employment history
- hobbies and recreational activities
- major lifetime achievements
- family and marriage
- retirement and social engagement.

Life Review Therapy

Life review therapy is a more structured intervention, with sessions planned ahead, mapping out life stages that will be covered. Life review therapy is an exceptionally effective intervention with older people living in the community and in residential care. This type of structured intervention is used mainly with older people who have depression. It is beneficial in improving the mood as it encourages older people to remember and review memories or past events.

Benefits of Reminiscence

If you are not yet convinced of the benefits of reminiscence, here are some more evidence-based findings. First, reminiscence helps us appreciate the challenges faced by older people in later life. It is truly remarkable to hear some of the stories from older people of the challenges they faced and how they overcame them. This can not only help with our own resilience but also theirs, as it builds on their character strengths, boosts confidence and increases self-esteem. Reminiscence makes a connection between a person's past, present and future and helps an individual transition through life stages. Further, reminiscence confirms a sense of unique identity and encourages feelings of self-worth which assists the process of life review. Lastly, reminiscence encourages open communication, aids assessment of present functioning and informs care plans. It helps to involve older people in any decision-making relating to their care plans, incorporating not only their physical health but also emotional wellbeing and lifestyle preferences.

Reminiscence and Depression

Research has shown that reminiscence with individuals who experience depression is particularly beneficial in both one on one settings and group sessions. Instrumental reminiscence encourages reminiscers to identify recollections of successful past problem-solving and skills which can help them overcome the challenges that they are currently facing.

For older adults with depression isolation is the common issue; they feel disconnected from their environment and peers. Reminiscence individually and even more so in a group setting can boost social engagement and improve clinical outcomes. It is common that depressed individuals tend to recall depressed memories. However, it's important not to assume their whole life has been sad. Their memories only reflect their current state and with some gentle guidance they can focus on happier times in their lives, which can be boosted with increased social interactions.

Reminiscence and Sensory Impairment

Often there is an assumption that sensory impairment will affect reminiscence and that it is simply too difficult to engage in such activity. However, individuals with sensory impairment perhaps need reminiscence the most. It is important to differentiate between sensory impairment acquired in late life and lifelong sensory impairment, such as individuals who have had language or hearing impairment since birth. In aged care, sensory impairment is common and many older people may have declining vision and hearing loss. Sometimes these individuals may experience low confidence, lack motivation, have low self-esteem and a fear of making fools of themselves or being a burden to others. Or, they may engage in maladaptive behaviours, which includes not using aids in fear of being perceived as being old and 'dumb'.

To incorporate reminiscence with older people it is important to put the person ahead of their disability. Think about the individual and their life experience rather than what has happened to their health and the impact this has on them. According to Butler (2004), there are three key principles when working with older people who have sensory impairment (and in my experience these will benefit the majority of older people). First, use brighter settings, increase lighting and do not sit in dark rooms. Second, use bigger images and writing where possible, enlarged images are very beneficial as well as handouts with fonts size 14 or larger. Third, use bold contrasting colours, it can help with reading and seeing materials. Try and use multi-sensory triggers, rather than relying on one sense alone as well as non-verbal and verbal communication skills, such as your body language, the tone of your speech and mannerisms.

Culturally Diverse Backgrounds

Reminiscence with those from culturally diverse backgrounds is powerful and can assist in learning about an individual's history, religion, values, beliefs, customs and traditions. It can also help you learn about cultural difference towards ageing, death and dying. As with any older person, the benefits of engaging in reminiscence with those from culturally diverse backgrounds are endless – it can encourage ethnic elders to share their recollections, develop memorabilia collections, keep culture alive, help to make services more responsive to a variety of needs and assist in overcoming myths and stereotypes.

Before engaging in reminiscence with individuals from culturally diverse backgrounds, it is important to research the particular culture so you can be sensitive when questioning. Careful listening to develop understanding about what it is like to grow old in a second homeland is also very important as is ethically sensitive reminiscence work, which can help to inform about differences of religion, ethnicity, age, gender, classes and status. Both individual and group work is effective, and in my experience group work in particular has been beneficial as individuals from culturally diverse backgrounds enjoy sharing stories from their upbringing and how they overcame challenges.

Reminiscence and Terminally Ill

When facing death, many people seek to find meaning in life. Therefore, in particular when working with people who are terminally ill it is important that they are being listened to and being reassured. Dying people may want to express their deepest feelings, admit past mistakes, make restitution, or even forgive themselves for actual or perceived mistakes, but may find it difficult to do so. Music in end of life care brings great comfort.

Incorporating reminiscence with an older person who is terminally ill is not necessarily challenging. The skills required for this include respecting the individual regardless of their disability and age, openly recognising and acknowledging grief and adjusting communication. If possible, use tangible and verbal reminders to encourage the recall of memories to assist in appreciating and celebrating the life lived and importantly provide continuing, respectful and appreciative support.

DIGGING DEEP

1. Do you often reminisce?

2. Why do older people enjoy talking about the 'good old days'?

3. Do you feel that sharing memories with older people would improve your relationship with them?

Part V

Integrated Collaboration

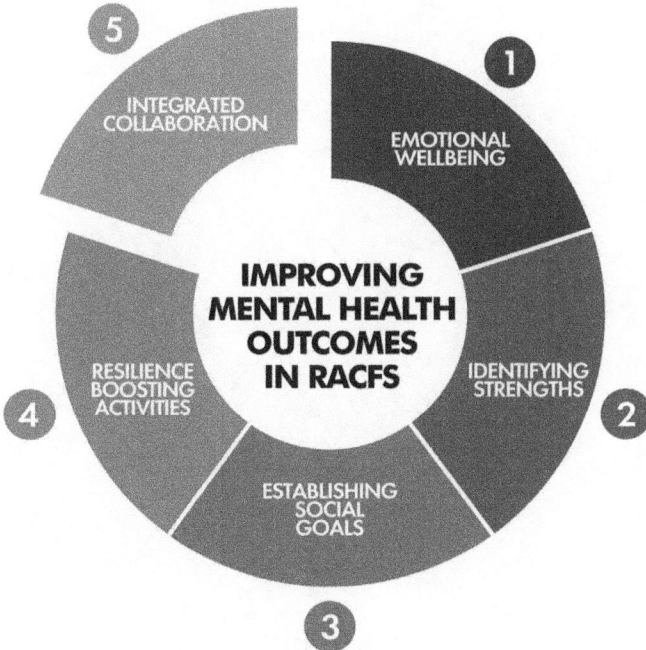

CHAPTER 10

Building Support Networks

Achieving positive and holistic outcomes in residential aged care facilities cannot be done in isolation. It requires a team effort, collaboration and open communication.

The older adults who are best adjusted to an aged care environment are usually the ones who have:

- a good support network
- open communication with their loved ones
- supportive and understanding care delivery from facility staff
- open and regular communication between all parties
- insight into their level of care needs
- a desire to maintain regular engagement with activities offered on site at the facility or within their local community.

Close bonds are often formed between caregiver and care recipient and this is something that needs to be acknowledged, as being both physically and psychologically present is essential. A good support network does not magically happen – it requires careful planning, attentive listening, timely response, day-to-day support and end-of-life care. Sometimes the older person only requires to be heard, rather than necessarily have something changed. Being able to talk through their worries or concerns allows them to better adjust and cope with changes and feel less isolated. And, changes are inevitable as we approach the end of life and the support we may require.

Over the years, I've visited many residential aged care facilities, and it is easy to observe the extent to which the aged care workforce are meeting the needs of older people, both when they are in good health and when their health is declining. This includes support with the initial adjustment right up to delivering end-of-life care. Yes, some people do die in facilities, either unexpectedly or because they chose to receive support in the facility rather than go into hospital, and those wishes in many instances can be met. Staff are trained in how to deliver end-of-life care and support. An older person facing the end of their life can feel more comfortable surrounded by familiar staff, in a familiar environment rather than being in a hospital setting. It is a human right to choose where we die and how we wish to be supported in our final days. For this reason, when an older person is admitted to an aged care facility there are usually forms to be completed about their choice of end-of-life care and the level of support and intervention they may wish to have, including if they wish to be resuscitated or not.

A Personal Insight

'In my decade of visiting aged care facilities I have only been involved in supporting two dying patients. Most deaths in my experience happened either outside of business hours, in hospital or the person was significantly

supported by their family that there was no need for a mental health professional to be involved as well. The two experiences that I have had, both during my pregnancies, were very different. They have both reminded me of the importance of effective teamwork and collaboration in supporting the older dying person.

The first instance was of an elderly client who was socially isolated. She was beautiful inside and out, someone I knew for a number of years prior to her death and who had a long history of late onset depression following her declining physical health and move to an aged care facility. She had one son who was adopted and rarely visited and a very supportive but extended family interstate. On the morning of the day when she passed away staff advised me that her health had declined and that I may wish to visit her. I entered her room and noted she was in bed, and was non-verbal at that stage but acknowledged my presence by squeezing my hand. Over the course of six hours, while I was in and out of the room and attending to other appointments, her health declined and she passed away in the afternoon. I am privileged that I was by her side when she died, as her main fear was of dying alone in an aged care facility. I remember holding her hand as she was taking her final breaths and also feeling the baby move in my belly. That was such a magical experience. Staff were in and out of the room, checking up every half an hour or so, as their schedule allowed. The death of this resident was around the time of a handover for the afternoon shift, so in nursing terms it was not the best time, not that you can really time the death.

The second death was more recent, and also an elderly female client who had a fall and hip surgery, however, once she returned to the facility her health never improved. This lady was travelling the world with her husband right up to when they were both admitted to an aged care facility. They shared with me that they had a big fight in a hotel room, as they were about to go on their overseas trip. The fight escalated to the point that they had intervention from hotel staff and police and subsequently, due to their declining cognitive abilities, they were hospitalised and moved to an aged care facility. Adjustment to living in the facility was difficult for them, as they were used to travelling, eating at fine dining restaurants and having great entertainment. Suddenly, they found themselves in a routine of 8am breakfast, midday lunch and 5pm dinner. Staff encouraged them to engage in activities and interact with other residents, however, their ability to do so was affected with their cognitive decline. When the wife was entering palliative care it all become too much for her husband. He did not wish to see her in that state and staff supported him in the loss that he was going through, whilst at the same time ensuring his wife was kept comfortable and free from pain. Her passing was quick and supported by two staff members on each side holding her hand and gently speaking with her. It was amazing to see staff caring so well for someone who was taking their final breaths.

What I didn't realise is that even after the person passes away the care does not stop. Carers attend to the deceased by washing the body and dressing the person before the funeral parlour collects the body. So, they need to be emotionally prepared to deal with the task, putting aside their own grief and loss associated with the death of a client, someone they would have had a close relationship with prior to the older person's death. This is a remarkable task to attend and something not often discussed outside of work hours. This is called workplace grief and loss.

Over the years I have delivered a number of sessions on workplace grief and loss at residential aged care facilities. Staff have attended seeking tips and advice on how to best cope after the resident passes away. This included supporting those who were present when the person passed away as well as those who may have turned up on a shift and another resident was in the same room. The key aspect of workplace grief and loss is understanding how we process loss in our lives and the strategies we use to gain a sense of closure. This improves our resilience and minimises the risk of burnout.'

An Older Person's Declining Health

It is inevitable that at some stage our health will decline and that we may no longer be as resilient, fit and vibrant as we were some time ago. It can be difficult to determine the cause of the decline and its permanency. Is this something that is likely to be reversed or is it part of the health condition that the older person has? How can staff and families support the older person in this process, ensuring that they encourage some type of pleasant activity that the older person may choose to engage in and are physically able to do so?

Adapting the approach to emotional wellbeing and activity levels is the key to successful adjustment. A similar concept needs to be implemented in late life, as it does when an individual slows down from high impact activities, such as bushwalking and hiking to walking on flat ground and to the lesser degree. Instead of stopping the activity completely, this is the time when the older person may require more support to meet their social and emotional needs. The adapted approach may include initially supporting the older person to be engaged in their local community, taking them to appointments outside the facility, to later on being able to meet social needs during briefer visits, pending on the health status of the older person, their energy levels and ability to engage in the visit. Some of the strategies may include taking them in a wheelchair outside to enjoy some time in the sun and fresh air instead of being indoors. This is also the time that family may be able to organise some special visits that the older person may wish to do, such as one more trip to the beach, a drive in the car or meal at their favourite restaurant. There have been occasions where the older person may even have a simple request, such as getting ice-cream from McDonald's!

'I know I will only leave this place in a box,' said James. This attitude to declining physical health and views of death and dying in residential care can be confronting for many older adults. In many instances,

they did not foresee that their health would decline in an unfamiliar environment nor that they would move into residential care. However, many older people will in fact die in residential care and their health will decline. This shifts the care delivered to the individual from focusing on prevention and active intervention to one where the focus is on keeping the older person free from pain and discomfort and working closely with health professionals, such as GPs and the palliative care team, when and if appropriate, to support the older person.

Declining resident heath can be difficult to accept for even the most resilient aged care workers, as there is no linear trend in how we all age and the decline that we are likely to experience. Some people decline quicker than others and they may have sudden setbacks in their health and prognosis. The uncertainty of the health decline can impact staff and their coping mechanisms, particularly if they formed a close bond with the older person. It is not uncommon for staff to return from holidays, or even after the weekend, and the older person's health has declined to a point where they have entered the end-of-life stage or passed away. In those instances it can be difficult to come on shift and find out that the client is no longer in the same health that they were in only few days earlier, or that they are in hospital without planned discharge or have passed away.

Over the years, many families have shared experiences of an older person passing away in the facility. For some, they had their family there to support them, but in many instances (statistically up to 40% of residents do not have visitors) the death can be a lonely experience with staff coming and going according to their roster and the dying client dealing with handover and staffing changes in the final moments of their lives. In those instances an allied health professional, chaplain or a manager may be supporting the older person if they are on site during that time. Having said that, there have been a number of occasions where the older person passed away peacefully in their sleep overnight without anyone beside them in those final moments. This is another type of death that can also impact the workers, as many find it difficult knowing that the older person died alone.

For those clients who have families who visit them and deliver support on site, it is not uncommon to spend significantly more time with the older person as their health declines. Sometimes families may stay overnight or take turns between relatives to ensure the older person is not alone if it is evident they are not likely to live for much longer. Families can help to create a peaceful environment for the older person in their room, playing soft music, holding the older person's hand and speaking gently with them. It is also an incredibly precious and personal time where staff respect the close bond between families and older people and do not intrude. In those instances, there can be disconnection between the grief experienced by the family and also the worker, who may wish to say their final goodbye to the older person whom they supported for a period of their stay at the facility.

Care Conferences

Care conferencing is the time when the older person's health and wellbeing is discussed between the older person, their family, facility and treating professionals. Care conferencing is usually conducted a couple of times per year, however it may be more frequent. Care conferencing is a helpful strategy to review the care the older person receives and if there are any strategies that can be implemented to assist with their health. It is also an opportunity for families to discuss any concerns they may have and opportunities to advocate for additional support and resources for the older person.

It is, however, not uncommon for the older person not to be involved in this important meeting. Sometimes the older person may not be able to engage in the meeting due to their health status or insight into support needs. In those instances their family will attend the conference alone. Sometimes families may require additional supports and information how to support their loved one and how to enhance the quality of their interactions with the older person, treating doctor and the facility. The process of supporting a loved one's transition to an aged care home can be overwhelming and uneasy. It is therefore important for the facility to ensure that the family is receiving the right support and guidance.

Multidisciplinary Collaboration

The term interdisciplinary suggests 'multi' which means more than one discipline. To achieve the best outcomes for the older person in residential care and in line with the older person's needs, it is important for the service provider to work in collaboration with a multidisciplinary team of health professionals. From the perspective of the aged care facility, this initially includes collaboration between clinical staff and leisure and lifestyle personnel to help the older person achieve their goals at the facility. The process also includes involving families and keeping them informed of the older person's changes in health and treatment, particularly if a person responsible has been identified.

There have been a number of instances where the older person can become upset if their next-of-kin is notified about an issue which they perceive to be trivial and irrelevant, such as putting on 2kg in a month or if the staff are concerned that the older person is eating too much sugar. In those instances the older person reports that they feel somewhat embarrassed and wished that the concern was discussed with them first before the phone call was made to their relative. Similarly, in some instances the person responsible may not in fact be emotionally close to the older person and they may perceive the monthly 'care update calls' to not be relevant or useful. It is important in those instances to discuss with the team the frequency and nature of routine updates and ensure that it is in line with the older person's preference and consent.

Many older people in residential care have chronic health conditions which require a multidisciplinary approach. For example, if they have type II diabetes, they may require reviews with:

- an endocrinologist to monitor their blood sugar levels
- a podiatrist to review circulation in their feet
- an eye specialist to review any damage to their eyes from glaucoma
- a dietitian to review dietary intake in line with relevant sugar content
- physiotherapist to review their activity levels and exercise in the facility.

DIGGING DEEP

1. What is the role of a support network for an older person?

2. Do you feel that some older people may have difficulty in identifying their support network and instead feel anger towards certain individuals due to their circumstances?

3. Do you feel that it is important for an older person to be present in their care conference?

CHAPTER 11

Involving
Families

Families of older adults in residential care play an important role in helping the older person adjust to the new environment. They provide background information and insight to the facility, which guides them in how to best support the older person. The provision of insight into personal preferences, likes and dislikes and individual characteristics can assist the aged care workforce to ensure that the older person's needs are met and minimise the risk of distress. This is particularly useful if the older person has cognitive changes or sensory impairments which impact their ability to express themselves. Families are commonly involved in the initial process of instigating the move to residential care, which includes assisting the older person to select the facility and completing all the necessary admission paperwork. Post move, families are involved on an ongoing basis with care planning and meeting the older person's social needs, by mitigating the frequency and level of contact in line with the needs of the older person and their own availability.

Often it is the families who instigate the move and facilitate the transition, recognising that the older person's level of care needs is higher than the support available for in-home care. The decision to move the older person into residential care can be difficult, particularly if the older person received a high level of support in their home and the family members feel stressed, tired and are experiencing burnout. The older person may lack insight into their care needs and be in denial about the increased level of support and their ability to cope in the home environment. Similarly, family members may find it difficult to recognise when their elderly relative's level of care needs has increased and how to broach the subject of supported accommodation without causing tension in the relationship. There can be negative connotations associated with the move and the perception from families that no matter what, the older person should stay in their own home. Unfortunately, this may not always be possible.

Decision-Making by Families

Often the children of older adults are appointed the authority to make decisions on behalf of the older person whose health is declining and who are no longer able to make their own decisions or manage financial affairs independently. The decision-making by families can range from having the power of attorney, being an enduring guardian or financial management. These types of appointments are typically formally appointed by legal representatives engaged by the older person prior to their health declining and help in determining the level of support and care needed as their health declines and they enter end-of-life care.

In recent years there has been an increased awareness about involving the older person in the decision-making process and ensuring that their views are considered even in instances where their capacity may be diminishing. This may include reviewing preferences of the older person prior to their deteriorating health and involving them in a reduced capacity in the process by adapting the communication style and reducing the information overload. This approach can ensure the older person's views and preferences are considered and accounted for and increase their involvement and sense of control in decision-making.

Acknowledging Emotional Needs in Families

Families go through their own journey and process of accepting that their loved one has moved into residential care. For some, the decision was made relatively easily, particularly if the older person has been acceptive of the move and has an insight into their increasing level of care needs and supports into the future. For other families, it may be a more difficult journey, where the older person's health may have suddenly declined and both the older person and their family may require additional support to accept the transition. A daughter whose mother moved into residential care shared in a family support session how she often needed some time in her car before and after visiting her mother at the facility. For some families it can be difficult to respond to the older person who may be asking to be discharged from care and to return to their own homes and for others they may have a sense of relief that their loved one is receiving the professional care and support they require in light of their declining physical health. Every family is unique and the ways in which they approach this process varies due to their own personal factors as well as the external environment and pressures.

It is not uncommon for relatives who provided care prior to the admission into the aged care facility to experience stress, burnout and psychological distress. At a conference some years ago, a study was discussed where the level of carer stress prior to admission into the aged care facility, during the admission and after the relative passed away was measured. The findings showed that the carer stress levels remained the same when the older person was in care and that it was only after the person passed away that the stress levels reduced. This suggests that placing a loved one in residential care is not necessarily seen as an 'offload' of care and that the relatives are still involved both physically and emotionally in caring for their loved one in supported accommodation. Further, these findings highlight the role that families play in supporting the older person and also the importance of recognising their own wellbeing needs on an ongoing basis.

Family members may require additional supports and coping skills to recognise their own emotional needs and to learn strategies in how to incorporate self-care after their loved one moves into the facility. This may include scheduling regular time off, mapping out visits to the facility and allowing time for the older person to adjust to the new environment by getting to know staff and programs on offer at the facility. There is no fast and hard rule as to how often the visits should take place or how long they should last. It is more important to ensure that the visits are fulfilling for both parties and that they are sustainable, rather than to cause additional stress and reduce the downtime that both parties may need to rest and rejuvenate.

Top 5 Facts About Me

This resource was developed to assist communication between the older person, their family and the facility. The concept behind the resource is to encourage families to prepare ahead for meetings with the facility or care reviews by documenting the type of information that may be useful to know about the older person and their preferences. The Top 5 Facts About Me is a simple task and the template can be found in Appendix 5.

Here is a sample of the type of information that can be filled in:

1   *Mum was always physically active and enjoyed playing tennis and walking. Please encourage her to attend morning exercise and provide reassurance if she appears to lack confidence about her physical strength.*

2   *Mum has never liked to drink coffee, please make sure you always offer her tea – not ask every day if she wants tea or coffee.*

3   *Every Thursday, Mum and I will go out of the facility for a drive. Please ensure she is showered and ready for 10am pick up.*

4   *Mum was a teacher and enjoys being in a group environment. Please encourage her to attend the discussion group.*

5   *Mum is a modest lady and she is embarrassed that she can no longer shower independently. Please try and distract her during this task by discussing another topic, such as cooking, to take her mind off the fact that she needs help with showering.*

Dealing with Challenges

Unfortunately, the move into an aged care home can also cause tension in some families. This may include disagreements about moving a loved one into care, where one party sees it as an essential step due to the older person's declining physical health while other family members are opposed to the move, arguing for the older person to remain living in their own home. Disagreements may also arise about the location of the home and if it is closer to one relative or another and the reasons for selecting a particular facility. This tension can impact the older person's adjustment to residential care as they navigate the new environment whilst trying to resolve family issues. Further, tensions may arise between family members during visits and this is an issue that may require additional strategies and support.

On the other hand, some families may have been estranged for a long period of time prior to the admission yet the estranged relative may be listed as the next of kin. In those instances the person responsible may not have insight into the older person's level of care needs and supports and may not be involved in the adjustment to the new environment. This can impact the older person's adjustment to the new environment and highlight their level of isolation and limited support network. Some years ago an elderly client often spoke affectionately about her adopted son who had very limited contact with her and would rarely visit. On one occasion the facility contacted the son to provide an update on his mother's health and to advise that she was depressed, his response was, *'What does she have to be depressed about?'*. Unfortunately, this feedback did not increase the level of his engagement and the lady passed away not having seen her son for over 18 months.

Working Collaboratively with Families

Teamwork between the older person, their family and the facility can be highly beneficial and mutually rewarding for all parties. For the older person, it can help achieve person-centred care, individualised help and support in line with their wishes and interests, through self-expression and advocacy from their loved ones. Assistance from families can be particularly beneficial if the older person's health is declining and they have difficulties in expressing themselves and their needs. For facilities, working closely with families can help them better understand the needs of the older person, taking the guesswork out of the equation with regards to support needs and the preference for service delivery. Good communication can assist the adjustment process to the new environment and help form a bond between the caregiver and care recipient. A good working relationship between the facility and the older person's family can further assist in promptly addressing any issues and concerns that may arise. Each party plays an important role in supporting the older person and their adjustment to the new environment and through collaboration and effective communication the best outcomes for the older person can be achieved.

For some relatives, it can be difficult to visit the facility and see the deterioration in their loved one's health. There have been several instances where an elderly couple moved into a facility and one of them passed away, with the other remaining in the facility. For some adult children the visits can be difficult, as they often think about the relative who passed away and cannot bring themselves to visit the facility, despite the fact that the living relative still calls the place their home. The aged care environment can be confronting for some individuals, seeing people in wheelchairs or in dementia units where it is evident that they have a high level of support needs.

Families play an important role in supporting the older person's adjustment to the aged care environment. However, it is important to note that families are often complex units and that the move to the facility may in fact highlight some longstanding tensions between individuals or cause a breakdown in relationships. This may be between siblings or between the older person and their children. There are various causes for these rifts including varying levels of insight into the care needs of the older person, supports available to prevent admission, financial concerns and the nature of the relationship before the decline in the older person's health. Therefore, it is important to be flexible when working with families and to avoid setting high expectations on individuals and their commitment. There will always be a varying level of commitment between individuals and how often they visit their loved one and keep in touch between visits. This could range from daily visits to visiting once a year. In some instances where the person has great difficulty adjusting at admission there have been examples of families spending the night at the facility or developing a visit schedule between family members. Some relatives may prefer to spend the entire time at the facility during the visit while others may prefer to pick up their loved one from outside the facility and take them for a drive or a meal out – often it is a combination of both.

DIGGING DEEP

1. How can families of older people in residential care be more involved in day-to-day activities?

2. What strategies do you feel could work in dealing with challenges?

3. What happens if the older person and their family do not agree on certain aspects of older person's care needs?

CHAPTER 12

Psychological Wellbeing for the Workforce

The focus of the previous chapters has been on factors associated with the wellbeing of older people in residential care. In this chapter the attention turns to workers and their own wellbeing needs, both during work hours and while off work – in particular, being able to switch off at the end of the work day.

Th workforce here, broadly recognises the role of care staff members, nurses, leisure and lifestyle personnel, allied health professionals, administrators, hospitality workers, cleaners and the impact of client interactions on their wellbeing. Each worker plays an important role in the lives of older people, forming bonds and connections while delivering support. It is therefore no surprise that many workers are affected by changes in client status and particularly the grief and loss associated with client death.

Emotional care is broadly defined as an ability to deliver support which is not focused on the physical needs of the care recipient. In many ways, emotional care in aged care can be seen as the core requirement of service delivery. A positive working relationship between client and worker is paramount and benefits both parties. However, if the two parties clash the rest of the care could be compromised. The client may not feel comfortable to receive assistance and likewise the worker may feel reluctant to attend to the client for fear of being judged. Similarly, if the worker is having personal issues it can be hard to come to work, mask their true feelings and deliver the services in a jovial manner. In the aged care sector it is difficult to hide away for the day and not interact with clients, something that is perhaps a bit easier in an office-based job. Being able to detach from true feelings can be challenging, particularly if personal issues are present and clients can pick up on worker's energy levels, non-verbal cues and demeanour to determine that something is not right. For many, it can be difficult to mask true feelings from the ones required in their role.

The findings from the Royal Commission into Aged Care (2019–2020) suggest that workers feel stressed and experience burnout on a regular basis. The feedback indicates that a number of older people are entering residential care later in life and staying at home in poor health as long as possible. Subsequently, an older person's stay in residential care is much shorter and therefore they may only come to the facility for a couple of weeks before they pass away. This affects the wellbeing of the workers who are dealing with death and dying on a far more frequent basis than before. If the older person is not approaching end-of-life care but they have a chronic disease which prevents them from staying in their own home, they are likely to experience stress and frustration at not being able to remain independent in the community. Some of those frustrations may be projected to the workers and result in unpleasant interactions, not because of the nature of the relationship between the two parties but rather due to the older person's difficulty accepting their health status and environmental change. Therefore, the aged care workforce needs to be well equipped with skills and strategies in not only recognising how to physically support the older person but also how to deliver emotional care, particularly if the older person has difficulty adjusting to their new environment.

Preventing Burnout

Supporting older adults who are emotionally unwell presents its own challenges.

What type of skills does a worker need to become emotionally stronger and resilient to deliver better care, and at the same time ensure their own emotions are in check? This may include possessing a high level of resilience, self-efficacy and self-care practices. Resilience tests one's ability to adapt to circumstance in their life while self-efficacy refers to an individual's belief about their own capacities including decision-making around how they handle certain situations both at work and at home. Self-care refers to the practice of taking action to preserve or improve one's own health and is highly individualised. For example, listening to music may be beneficial to some individuals whilst playing golf is more rewarding for others. Individuals with low self-efficacy, resilience and irregular self-care practices are more prone to experiencing higher levels of stress and burnout.

Stress is defined as a state of mental or emotional strain or tension resulting from adverse or demanding circumstances. Everyone experiences stress to some extent, however the cumulative effects of stress can be detrimental to an individual and their wellbeing and can lead to burnout. Burnout is defined as a chronic physical and emotional exhaustion. In addition to burnout, individuals may also experience an inability to switch off at the end of the day, depersonalisation of issues experienced at work, compassion fatigue (where they experience tiredness in delivering compassionate care), occupational stress and psychological workplace injury. Workers may not know where to turn for support or how to improve their own coping skills and subsequently experience unpleasant symptoms for far too long. This can lead to reduced job satisfaction and increased possibility of wanting to change jobs or quit working in the aged care sector all together.

Approaches to Coping Styles

Everyone copes with stress in a different way using their own strategies. However, there are two coping styles adapted by humans which are broadly defined as adaptive and maladaptive. Adaptive coping strategies generally involves addressing the issues as soon as they arise, debriefing after a difficult day at work, recognising the response to stress and engaging in energy boosting activities that are enjoyable. This may include going for a walk, talking to a friend, spending time in a garden or watching a movie. These strategies are aimed to prevent adverse effects on the body, such as changes in sleeping habits, nutrition and stress levels. Individuals who engage in an adaptive coping style regularly communicate with management about events which have affected them, look for opportunities to debrief with peers and seek out strategies which are good for their wellbeing.

Maladaptive coping strategies are the opposite of adaptive strategies. This includes approaches which do not assist in dealing with the problem directly and avoid addressing the cause and the effects of the issue. Maladaptive coping strategies are unhelpful, as they do not teach the individual how to problem-solve and usually involve the use of alcohol and other drugs to supress true emotions and escape problems. Sometimes individuals may think that avoiding the discussion of the problem will make it go away quicker and cause less stress. However, not discussing the psychological impact of events and problem-solving can lead to more suffering.

Worker Wellbeing

Everyone has good and bad days, it is part of being human and juggling work and life balance. However, some individuals may experience higher levels of stress and more bad than good days. In many cases it may not be possible or practical to suggest, *'pull yourself together'* or to *'shake off'* some feelings and these symptoms could be suggestive of an underlying mental health condition, such as anxiety and/or depression. It is estimated by Beyond Blue (2020), one of the key mental health organisations in Australia, that over 2 million Australians currently live with anxiety and 1 million with depression. Further, on average more than eight people in Australia take their own lives every day, six of whom are men. Early detection of emotional changes and seeking support is crucial in reducing the prevalence of mental health conditions and reducing the risk of suicide.

The number of people seeking support appears to be growing at a rapid rate, with around half of those with a mental health condition now getting treatment from a professional (Beyond Blue, 2020). While depression rates are more common in females than in males, suicide rates are far higher in men. It is important for individuals who have persistent low mood and stress to speak to their GP about the symptoms and seek appropriate support. People of all ages, backgrounds and cultures are asking themselves, *'How can I feel better?'* and *'Will I feel like this for the rest of my life?'*. The good news is that with appropriate treatment, symptoms of depression and anxiety can be improved.

Resilience

Resilience is how well a person can adapt to the events in their life and is one of the keys to life satisfaction. Unlike your eye colour and height, resilience is a skill which can be built upon throughout life. There are a number of strategies to boost resilience which can be learned and practised on a regular basis.

Researchers suggest that resilience is underpinned with four key factors which are:

- your mental health status
- the practice of mindfulness
- your coping style
- your level of self-efficacy.

What is important to note from this list is that most of the factors can be taught – from the type of coping style implemented if issues arise to increasing self-efficacy and confidence at work and the practice of mindfulness. Even with the mental health status, getting appropriate treatment and support can improve an individual's wellbeing and resilience outcomes.

As covered earlier in Chapter 7, mindfulness is a form of meditation which improves your ability to be present in the moment. The techniques offered in Chapter 7 for older people can also be practised by the workforce, in particular, relaxation breathing, the body scan and recreational activities such as exercise, art therapy and relaxation. These techniques can take as little as five minutes each day or hours, depending on your schedule. However, research has shown that it is far more effective to engage in activities on a regular basis, such as short bursts of relaxation, rather than to put it off and only do it once in a blue moon. Using an adaptive coping style and problem-solving through difficulties will boost resilience, as will an improved perception of your own abilities and skills.

The important task for many who work in aged care is to identify a suitable time to work on their resilience. At an organisational level this may include discussing opportunities for an informal debrief and handover time, organising debriefs after difficult situations, regularly facilitating team building activities and ensuring workers understand and are encouraged to speak with their managers about any difficulties. For some, it may require a short break after dealing with a challenging situation, taking time off work or regularly scheduling holidays. Practising mindfulness at work through improved systems can help to deal with sudden and unexpected challenges as well as those anticipated which cannot be avoided. Providing information to workers about access to counselling and support is another strategy which can be arranged at an organisational level. Some aged care providers have Employee Assistance Programs in place, however, staff may not be aware of how to access this service.

On a more personal note, there are other strategies that can assist with reducing stress and boosting resilience. This may include using problem-solving with pen and paper, as shown in Chapter 7. Listing all the pros and cons of a situation and different ways to address the problem on paper can be helpful for many. Similarly, managing time using a diary or planner can also help you schedule in regular exercise, relaxation activities and holiday planning. Talking to a trusted friend or family member about any issues that may arise can be helpful, especially if you feel stuck about decisions you need to make. Lastly, engaging in light physical activity and relaxation techniques, or a combination of both through a yoga session can do wonders for your health and wellbeing.

DIGGING DEEP

1. What strategies do you use to minimise the risk of burnout?

2. Do you regularly engage in self-care strategies?

3. Do you feel that the aged care workforce needs more support and training in how to embed resilience into their day-to-day lives?

References

Australian Bureau of Statistics. (2008). *National Survey of Mental Health and Wellbeing: Summary of Results* (p 27). Retrieved from https://www.abs.gov.au/ausstats/abs@.nsf/mf/4326.0

Australian Bureau of Statistics. (2019). Australia's leading causes of death, 2018.

Australian Bureau of Statistics. Retrieved from https://www.abs.gov.au/ausstats/abs@.nsf/productsbytopic/47E19CA15036B04BCA2577570014668B?OpenDocument

Australian Institute of Health and Welfare [AIHW]. (2017). Australia's welfare 2017: in brief. *Canberra Australian Institute of Health and Welfare.* Retrieved from https://www.aihw.gov.au/reports/australias-welfare/australias-welfare-2017-in-brief/contents/ageing-and-aged-care

Australian Institute of Health and Welfare [AIHW]. (2019). Admissions into aged care. *Canberra Australian Institute of Health and Welfare.* Retrieved from https://www.gen-agedcaredata.gov.au/Topics/Admissions-into-aged-care

Bagley, H., Cordingley, L., Burns, A., Mozley, C. G., Sutcliffe, C., Challis, D., & Huxley, P. (2000). Recognition of depression by staff in nursing and residential homes. *Journal of Clinical Nursing, 9*(3), 445-450. doi: 10.1046/j.1365-2702.2000.00390.x

Butler, S. 2004. *Usher 2: How is it for You?* Sense, London

Byrne, G. J., Pachana, N., Goncalves, D., Arnold, E., King, R., & Keat, K. (2010). Psychometric properties and health correlates of the Geriatric Anxiety Inventory in Australian community-residing older women. *Aging & Mental Health, 14*(3), 247-254. doi: 10.1080/13607861003587628

Cherniack, E. P., & Cherniack, A. R. (2014). The benefit of pets and animal-assisted therapy to the health of older individuals. *Current gerontology and geriatrics research, 2014*, 623203. https://doi.org/10.1155/2014/623203

Christensen, H. (2001). What cognitive changes can be expected with normal ageing? *Australian and New Zealand Journal of Psychiatry*, 35, 768-775.

Davison, T., McCabe, M., Knight, T., & Mellor, D. (2012). Biopsychosocial Factors Related to Depression in Aged Care Residents. *Journal of Affective Disorders, 142*(1–3), 290-296. doi: http://dx.doi.org/10.1016/j.jad.2012.05.019

Dementia Australia, 2020, Help Sheets, Retrieved from https://www.dementia.org.au/resources/help-sheets#Your-Brain-Matters

Dols, A., Kupka, R.W., van Lammeren, A., Beekman, A.T., Sajatovic, M., & Stek, M.L. (2013). The prevalence of late life mania: a review. Bipolar Disorders 2014: 16: 113– 118.

Eyers, K., Parker, G., & Brodaty, T. (2012). *Managing Depression Growing Older*. Sydney: Allen & Unwin.

Farrow, M., & Ellis, K. Physical activity for brain health and fighting dementia. [Canberra]: Alzheimer's Australia, http://www.fightdementia.org.au/common/files/NAT/YBMPaper36_webfinal.pdf

Feldman, D. C. (1994). The Decision to Retire Early: A Review and Conceptualization. *The Academy of Management Review, 19*(2), 285–311. Retrieved from www.jstor.org/stable/258706

Fiske, A., Wetherell, J. L., & Gatz, M. (2009). Depression in older adults. *Annual review of clinical psychology, 5*, 363–389. https://doi.org/10.1146/annurev.clinpsy.032408.153621

Gibson, F. (2011). Reminiscence and Life Story Work: A Practical Guide. Jessica Kingsley Publishers, London.

Henderson, A., Jorm, A., Mackinnon, A., Christenson, H., Scott, L., Korten, A., & Doyle, C. (1994). A survey of dementia in the Canberra population: Experience with ICD-10 and DSM-III-R criteria. *Psychological Medicing, 24*(2), 473–482. doi:10.1017/S0033291700027446

Kerr, J., Marshall, S., Godbole, S., Neukam, S., Crist, K., Wasilenko, K., Golshan, S., & Buchner, D. (2012). The relationship between outdoor activity and health in older adults using GPS. *International journal of environmental research and public health, 9*(12), 4615–4625. https://doi.org/10.3390/ijerph9124615

Magaard, J. L., Seeralan, T., Schulz, H., & Brütt, A. L. (2017). Factors associated with help-seeking behaviour among individuals with major depression: A systematic review. *PloS one, 12*(5), e0176730. https://doi.org/10.1371/journal.pone.0176730

Murphy, B., Bugeja, L., Pilgrim, J., & Ibrahim, J. (2018). Suicide among nursing home residents in Australia: A national population based retrospective analysis of medico legal death investigation information. *International Journal of Geriatric Psychiatry, 33*, 786–796. https://doi.org/10.1002/gps.4862

National Ageing Research Institute. (2009). Depression in older age: a scoping study. Final Report. Melbourne: National Ageing Research Institute.

Olesen, S., & Berry, H. (2011). Community participation and mental health during retirement in community sample of Australians. *Aging and Mental Health, 15*(2), 186-197. https://doi.org/10.1080/13 607863.2010.501053

Pettit, S., Qureshi, A., Lee, W., Stirzaker, A., Gibson, A., Henley, W., & Byng, R. (2017). Variation in referral and access to new psychological therapy services by age: an empirical quantitative study. *British Journal of General Practice, 67* (660):453-459, e453-e459. DOI: 10.3399/ bjgp17X691361

Ribe A., Laursen T., & Charles M. (2015), Long-term risk of dementia in persons with schizophrenia: a Danish population-based cohort study. *JAMA Psychiatry, 72,* 1095–1101.

Stephan, Y., Fouquereau, E., & Fernandez, A. (2008). The relation between self-determination and retirement satisfaction among active retired individuals. *The International Journal of Aging and Human Development, 66*(4), 329–345. https://doi.org/10.2190/AG.66.4.d

Tampi, R. R., Young, J., Hoq, R., Resnick, K., & Tampi, D. J. (2019). Psychotic disorders in late life: a narrative review. *Therapeutic advances in psychopharmacology, 9*, 2045125319882798. doi. org/10.1177/2045125319882798

Tiwari S. C. (2013). Loneliness: A disease?. *Indian journal of psychiatry*, *55*(4), 320–322. doi.org/10.4103/0019-5545.120536

Tkach, C., & Lyubomirsky, S. (2006). How Do People Pursue Happiness? Relating Personality, Happiness-Increasing Strategies, and Well-Being. *J Happiness Stud,* 7, 183–225. https://doi.org/10.1007/s10902-005-4754-1

Uncapher, H., & Areán, P. A. (2000). Physicians are less willing to treat suicidal ideation in older patients. *Journal of the American Geriatrics Society, 48*(2), 188–192. doi.org/10.1111/j.1532-5415.2000.tb03910.x

Whiteford, H. A., Buckingham, W. J., Harris, M. G., Burgess, P. M., Pirkis, J. E., Barendregt, J. J., & Hall, W. D. (2014). Estimating treatment rates for mental disorders in Australia. *Australian Health Review, 38*, 80–85.

World Health Organisation. (2011, October). Retrieved from https://www.who.int/ageing/publications/global_health.pdf

World Health Organisation. (2017). Global action plan on the public health response to dementia 2017–2025. Retrieved from https://www.who.int/mental_health/neurology/dementia/action_plan_2017_2025/en/

Appendix 1

Planning Each Day

Each day it is important to factor in one of the four things – what will it be for you today?	
1. USEFUL	
2. ACTIVE	
3. INTELLECTUAL	
4. PLEASURABLE	

Appendix 2

Curating Social Goals

Sample Plan

	Task	Notes
STEP 1 →	Identify five enjoyable activities.	Enjoyable Activity 1 Enjoyable Activity 2 Enjoyable Activity 3 Enjoyable Activity 4 Enjoyable Activity 5
STEP 2 →	What are the client's top three strengths? (for example physical health, memory, good support network).	Strength 1 Strength 2 Strength 3
STEP 3 →	What are the five activities that the client is most interested in and physically able to do?	1. 2. 3. 4. 5.

	Task	Notes
STEP 4 →	*Considering the above and current environment, what are the three activities that the client is most passionate about?*	*Activity 1* *Activity 2* *Activity 3*

STEP 5
 	
→
	Based on the answers in Step 4, what can we establish as SMART goals which are achievable in the next four weeks?
	
	SMART Goals
	
	  • *Simple*
	  • *Measurable*
	  • *Achievable*
	  • *Realistic*
	  • *Timely*
		Goal 1
		Goal 2

STEP 6 →	*What are the goals that the client could engage in on a weekly basis? How about monthly goals?*	*Weekly Social Goal* *Monthly Social Goal*

Review	*Plan Review*	*Please Circle*
		  • *Weekly*
		  • *Monthly*
		  • *Bimonthly*
		  • *Quarterly*

Appendix 3

What Works for Emotional Wellbeing in Older People?

Here is a summary of what works for emotional wellbeing in older people in residential care settings.

Key	
?	There isn't enough evidence
✓	There is some evidence
✓✓	There is substantial evidence
✓✓✓	There is significant evidence

	Wellbeing	Anxiety	Depression
Physical activity			
• Exercise	✓✓✓	✓	✓✓
• Gardening and nature-assisted therapy	✓	?	✓
• Tai Chi and qigong	✓✓	?	?
• Yoga	✓	?	✓
Relaxation			
• Massage	✓✓	✓✓	?
• Meditation	✓✓	✓	?
Sensory stimulation			
• Aromatherapy	✓✓	✓✓	✓
• Snoezelen	✓	✓	✓
Music and arts			
• Art therapy and craft	✓	?	✓
• Music and singing	✓✓✓	✓✓✓	✓✓✓
Social activities			
• Animal and pet therapy	✓✓	?	✓✓
• Men's sheds	✓	✓	✓
Reflection			
• Life review	✓✓✓	?	✓✓✓
• Prayer and spiritual counselling	✓	?	✓
• Simple reminiscence	✓✓✓	?	✓✓✓

Quality of life approaches			
• Behavioural activation and pleasant events	✓✓✓	?	✓✓✓
• Person-centred care	✓✓	✓	?
Interventions delivered by mental health professionals			
• Cognitive behavioural therapy	✓✓	✓	✓✓
• Life review therapy	✓✓✓	✓	✓✓
• Mindfulness-based approaches	✓	?	✓

Appendix 4

Exercise Certificate

CONGRATULATIONS _____ (NAME) _____

Residential Aged Care Facility recognises you have attended

50
EXERCISE SESSIONS

KEEP UP THE GREAT WORK!

Appendix 5

Top 5 Facts About Me

Top 5 is a simple activity where, in consultation with your loved one who is entering care, you list the five most important facts about them. The information can be very useful for aged care staff to better know your loved one and help to support their adjustment to residential care. You don't need to order them in priority, list them as they come to your mind. For example, *'Mum loves to sit near a window where she can watch the birds in the tree,'* or *'Dad loves watching movies and trivia, please include him in those activities'.*

So, what are the top five facts about your loved one? Note them here:

1	
2	
3	
4	
5	

Appendix 6

Welcome Booklet for New Residents

Coming to a residential care facility can create mixed feelings for individuals. For some, there is a sense of relief that they no longer need to do the household chores. While for others, it creates unpleasant and unhappy feelings about not being able do some things and perhaps having to sell their home and dispose of personal belongings. Regardless of your circumstances, you are likely to feel overwhelmed by the experience. This is a normal part of adjustment and in time you will find that you will 'just get used to it'.

By now you have probably completed a number of questionnaires with staff about your medical and physical needs as well as your interests. We suggest that you do not be disheartened as it is natural to take some time to join in the activities. Please, review the program and give it a go. This is a way to get to know people and you may enjoy taking part in a new activity!

We all like to spend some time alone when we can and this is also perfectly normal. It is always nice to have a fine balance between mixing with people and spending some time alone.

If you are not happy with how something is done you need to let someone on the staff know your preferences. The staff are trained in carrying out activities in a manner which assists the resident to maintain and enhance their self-esteem and self-worth. You can also complete a feedback form which you will find at the front desk. It is important that all the residents are treated with respect and dignity and that the residents also treat staff with equal values.

Again, welcome to this facility and we look forward to getting to know you.

Best wishes,

The Residents

About
the Author

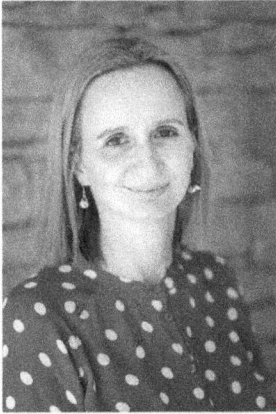

With a high level of compassion for the elderly, Dr **Julie Bajic Smith**, Registered Psychologist, embarked on a clinical and research adventure to learn more about older adults and their needs in residential care. Her journey included supporting hundreds of older adults and their families and training the workforce which encouraged her to write *Beyond the Reluctant Move*. Julie is a clinician who has completed postgraduate research on the relationship of mental health and ageing. She has trained postgraduate students and mental health professionals on the unique needs of older adults in residential aged care. Julie is sought after as a speaker at industry conferences and is dedicated to beating the myth that depression and dementia are a normal part of ageing.

Acknowledgements

The first draft of this book was based on my experience of working with over 300 older adults across several aged care facilities in Sydney, Australia. I would like to say a huge thank you to all the residents and their families for having so much trust and faith in my services, and for the constant feedback that you have given me over the years.

To aged care workers, team leaders, managers and service providers, thank you for your insight, collaboration and input. A very special thank you to all the amazing professionals who were interviewed for the Voice of Aged Care Podcast. Your insight and feedback about various strategies you implement to improve the wellbeing of older people in residential care are admirable.

My family and friends have continued to be a constant support of love and encouragement. A loving thank you to my husband, Justin, and children Hazel and Henry.

Finally, I would also like to say thank you to the hundreds of people who work in aged care and support older people who have taken the time to write to me and provide feedback on my podcast, training programs and their experience in incorporating techniques I suggested. Your constant feedback has been very important to me, and your loving supportive messages, mean more to me than you will ever know. A special thanks and love to you all.

How I can help

Julie is available for organisational consultations, training and support to improve mental health outcomes in residential aged care facilities. Julie's mission is to reduce the prevalence of mental health conditions across home care and residential aged care environment.

Workshop: Enhancing Emotional Wellbeing in Late Life – Practical Strategies

This 6-hour workshop is for anyone who supports older adults with declining physical health and is an extension of the principles covered in *Beyond the Reluctant Move* book. Learn the practical tools to implement strategies into the delivery of daily care. Program is delivered through e-Learning, however for some organisations a group booking can be facilitated on site.

Module 1 – Emotional Wellbeing
Module 2 – Identifying Strengths
Module 3 – Establishing Social Goals
Module 4 – Resilience Boosting Activities
Module 5 – Integrated Collaboration

Wellness Group Program – Building Strengths and Resilience

This award-winning program has been delivered to over 1000 older adults in residential settings and is set up to be licensed to aged care providers throughout Australia. Licensing involves Julie training a small group of aged care staff to run the sessions using Wise Care materials (session plan, facilitator background information on the topic and participant handouts). Facilitators are provided with regular and ongoing mentoring and support. The program consists of eight modules delivered four times per year (covers content for 32 weeks in a calendar year).

Guide for Families: Practical guide to support transition to residential aged care available electronically and in hard copy.

For more information about how Julie can assist your organisation please visit wisecare.com.au

www.ingramcontent.com/pod-product-compliance
Lightning Source LLC
Chambersburg PA
CBHW031124020426
42333CB00012B/221